AIDS and Civil Society

AIDS and Civil Society

India's Learning Curve

EDITED BY

RADHIKA RAMASUBBAN

BHANWAR RISHYASRINGA

Centre for Social and Technological Change, Mumbai

RAWAT PUBLICATIONS

Jaipur · New Delhi · Bangalore · Hyderabad · Guwahati

ISBN 81-7033-946-4

Reprinted 2010

Published by
Prem Rawat for Rawat Publications
Satyam Apts., Sector 3, Jawahar Nagar, Jaipur 302 004 (India)
Phone: 0141 265 1748 / 7006 Fax: 0141 265 1748
E-mail: info@rawatbooks.com
Website: www.rawatbooks.com

New Delhi Office
4858/24, Ansari Road, Daryaganj, New Delhi 110 002
Phone: 011-23263290

Also at Bangalore, Hyderabad and Guwahati

Typeset by Rawat Computers, Jaipur
Printed at Chaman Enterprises, New Delhi

Contents

SECTION THREE
Raising Awareness about Sexuality

SECTION FOUR
HIV/AIDS and Women in Prostitution

SECTION FIVE
HIV/AIDS as a Human Rights Issue and Men Who Have Sex with Men

SECTION SIX
Legal Approaches to HIV/AIDS

Preface

Nearly twenty years into the HIV/AIDS epidemic in India, the Indian public is yet to be drawn into the HIV/AIDS sector as well-informed and active participants in the vital public interest issues that HIV/AIDS has thrown up. Among the most obvious issues are: sexuality education for the young, citizenship rights for hitherto stigmatised minority communities, respect for social diversity including sexual diversity, the human right to education and information on means of self-protection against incurable and fatal diseases such as HIV/AIDS and, in the event of contracting such an infection, the right to be treated with dignity and respect on the basis of equality with other citizens. Beneath the surface of these, however, seethe the much larger and complex issues of social, economic and gender-based inequalities and disadvantage, oppressive cultural values and beliefs, and irrational fears and stigmas that plague our society. HIV/AIDS has also highlighted women and young people as those who are most vulnerable due to the above forces. And it has put responsibility on the shoulders of men to examine their own roles – and notions of masculinity – in abetting this vulnerability.

But how many even among educated Indians in urban areas really know what HIV/AIDS is all about? And of those who believe they know something about the disease, how many associate it with much more than public controversies about numbers of HIV positive people in the country, condom distribution drives, or unsafe blood transfusions? Today, the most public face of the epidemic consists of widespread confusion about the most elementary aspects of sexuality, a misplaced interpretation of the risks of HIV transmission in terms of sexual morality, and the ghettoisation and stigmatisation of positive people and those working to improve their lot.

Admittedly, there are few sources of cogent information about HIV/AIDS that the public has access to. Public messages warning people to 'Prevent AIDS' tend to be drab, simplistic, and often confusing and contradictory. Media stories of HIV/AIDS prevalence or of instances of victimisation of HIV positive persons veer towards sensationalism. Media publicity for celebrity endorsements of HIV/AIDS prevention efforts favours a focus on the celebrities rather than the problem. All of these make HIV/AIDS appear as 'something that happens to other people', and none give citizens any clues about the real issues involved. The fact is that, theoretically, everyone is at risk of HIV/AIDS. But everyone can also protect themselves and others from acquiring it through informed action.

One way in which citizens can learn more about the HIV/AIDS problem in the country – and the promises for and obstacles to its control – is to acquaint themselves with the complex contexts within which HIV/AIDS interventions and innovations are taking place. The agencies leading these interventions are non-governmental organisations or NGOs – organisations that are voluntarily set up by individuals to perform self-help or socially useful roles – which have been consistently and constructively involved in tackling HIV/AIDS at the grassroots level ever since the onset of the epidemic.

This book brings out for the first time an inside view of NGO-led HIV/AIDS intervention efforts on the ground. It focuses on six NGO interventions that have been at the cutting edge of efforts to combat the epidemic since the earliest days of the virus' appearance in the country. Starting off independently, led by professional individuals who gave up more lucrative career alternatives in favour of NGO activism and who chose to work in the HIV/AIDS arena at a time when every step was new ground to be broken, these NGOs have evolved and endured in the face of considerable odds. Today, nearly all of them are considered cases of 'best practices' in the field of HIV/AIDS intervention, and have spawned several others like themselves, and are part of larger networks of HIV/AIDS organisations that interact with and learn from each other.

There are several NGOs in the country doing excellent and dedicated work in the HIV/AIDS sector, and we cannot pretend to have made a representative selection out of them. The selection of case studies included in this book is arbitrary. What we do offer the reader here is a glimpse into six areas that have a unique relationship to the HIV/AIDS epidemic in India: treatment and care of positive people, prevention education at the workplace, sexuality education, women in prostitution, men who have sex with men, and legal approaches to issues raised by HIV/AIDS. The fact also is that in all of these frontiers, the NGOs in this book have been among the pioneers, and have been successful in developing both coherent conceptual approaches and practical intervention programmes.

There are six sections in the book, corresponding to the six areas in which the NGOs work. Each section begins with a short overview by the editors that lays out the principal issues pertaining to that particular area of the HIV/AIDS epidemic. These are not necessarily state-of-the-art accounts, but are meant to contextualise the individual case studies for the benefit of the reader. Following every overview is the case study itself.

We are grateful to Anand Grover, Anjali Gopalan, Daisy Dharmaraj, Jude Stephens, Meena Seshu, Radhika Chandiramani and Suniti Solomon for their contributions to the book. It is hard for NGOs who have to constantly strategise in response to daily practical challenges and crises – relating to people who are at the depths of despair, advocating their own respective causes, continuously crafting their organisations' growth paths in the light of changes taking place around them, seeking to achieve financial sustainability over the long term – to additionally have to cope with researchers who prod them to take time off to reflect on their experiences, not only their successes but more importantly their failures. That all of them responded to our initial request with a resounding yes; that they repeatedly reiterated their commitment to self-introspection through the many months when other exigencies consumed them and the book got interminably delayed and looked like it might never get done; and that they welcomed us to their project areas, talked to us at length about their work, shared their documentation, and willingly worked with us in a final spurt of energy to produce this joint effort, is a testimony to their sincerity of purpose.

Our thanks are also due to Shaleen Rakesh and A.K. Ganesh for useful discussions. We owe special thanks to Shireen Jejeebhoy and Priya Mutalik Desai for reading the manuscript and offering constructive suggestions. The usual disclaimers apply. We are indebted to Karen Smith, who edited the manuscript with great care and made available her quilt creation – Tumbling Blocks – for the book's cover design. Made from various and disparate scraps of fabric patchworked together into a unifying design, the quilt is symbolic of how diverse entities, when brought together by a vision of a whole, can create a thing of great beauty and value.

The idea of a book on HIV/AIDS interventions emerged out of a dialogue with Geeta Misra who prepared the early ground for it. We are grateful to her and to Roshmi Goswami for their sustained interest. The Ford Foundation was one of the earliest agencies to foresee the importance of supporting NGOs in HIV/AIDS interventions. Much of the work by the NGOs in this book, too, has benefitted from this support. We wish to acknowledge the role played by the Ford Foundation in the preparation of this book. Our final thanks go to Rawat Publications for their interest in the book's theme.

If this book can draw in readers as active supporters of worthy intervention efforts, or even as empathetic well-wishers of those who suffer on account of the disease, or at the very least prompt readers to introspect and examine their own latent prejudices, it will have played a useful role.

Radhika Ramasubban
Bhanwar Rishyasringa

Abbreviations

AIDS	:	Acquired Immunodeficiency Syndrome
AMTC	:	Affordable Medicines and Treatment Campaign
ART	:	Anti-Retroviral Therapy
ARV	:	Anti-Retroviral
CBO	:	Community-Based Organisation
CHETNA	:	Centre for Health Education Training and Nutrition Awareness
CII	:	Confederation of Indian Industry
CREA	:	Creating Resources for Empowerment in Action
DFID	:	Department for International Development
DOTS	:	Directly Observed Treatment Scheme
DMSC	:	Durbar Mahila Samanwaya Committee
ESIS	:	Employees State Insurance Scheme
HIV	:	Human Immunodeficiency Virus
HIV+	:	HIV positive
IDU	:	Intravenous Drug User
ILO	:	International Labour Organisation
INP+	:	Indian Network of Positive People
IPC	:	Indian Penal Code

LCHAU	:	Lawyers Collective HIV/AIDS Unit
MSM	:	Men who have Sex with Men
NACO	:	National AIDS Control Organisation
NGO	:	Non-Governmental Organisation
NMP+	:	Maharashtra Network of Positive People
MIC	:	Methyl Isocyanate
PEP	:	Post Exposure Prophylaxis
PREPARE	:	PREPARE India Rural Reconstruction and Disaster Response Service
PMTCT	:	Prevention-of-Mother-to-Child-Transmission
PIL	:	Public Interest Litigation
PLWHA	:	People Living with HIV/AIDS
RTIs	:	Reproductive Tract Infections
SANGRAM	:	Sampada Grameen Mahila Sanstha
SIDA	:	Swedish International Development Authority
STDs	:	Sexually Transmitted Diseases
STIs	:	Sexually Transmitted Infections
TARSHI	:	Talking About Reproductive and Sexual Health Issues
TB	:	Tuberculosis
TNSACS	:	Tamil Nadu State AIDS Control Society
TRIPS	:	Trade-Related Intellectual Property System
UNDP	:	United Nations Development Programme
VAMP	:	Veshya AIDS Mukabla Parishad
VDRL	:	Venereal Disease Research Laboratory Slide Test
WEG	:	Worker Education Group
WHO	:	World Health Organisation
WTO	:	World Trade Organisation
YRG CARE	:	Y.R. Gaitonde Centre for AIDS Research and Education

Contributors

ANAND GROVER is the Director of the Lawyers Collective HIV/AIDS Unit, Mumbai and New Delhi, and a practising advocate in the Bombay High Court.

The Lawyers Collective HIV/AIDS Unit provides legal aid and allied services for people affected by HIV/AIDS. Its main objective is to protect and promote the fundamental rights of persons living with HIV/AIDS, who have been denied their rights in areas such as health care, employment, terminal dues like gratuity and pension, and marital rights relating to maintenance and custody and housing. The Unit initiates public interest litigation on issues like the right to marry, confidentiality, access to health care, safe blood supply, and quacks. It also conducts workshops on legal and ethical issues relating to HIV/AIDS for people living with HIV/AIDS, lawyers, judges, health care providers and NGOs.

The Lawyers Collective HIV/AIDS Unit,
Programme Management Unit,
7/10 Botawalla Building, 2nd Floor,
Horniman Circle, Fort, Mumbai 400023.
Tel: 022-2267 6213/9
Fax: 022-270 2563
E-mail: aidslaw@vsnl.com
Website: www.lawyerscollective.org

ANJALI GOPALAN is the Executive Director of Naz Foundation (India) Trust, New Delhi.

The Naz Foundation (India) Trust is an HIV/AIDS service organisation working on issues of prevention and care. Their programmes include working with men who have sex with men, training and advocacy, women's sexual health, peer education in colleges, outpatient clinic services, home-based care, and a care home for orphan children and abandoned women living with HIV.

The Naz Foundation (India) Trust,
A-86 East of Kailash,
New Delhi 110065.
Telefax: 011-2691 0499/51325042
E-mail: nazindia@bol.net.in

DAISY DHARMARAJ was Founder-Director of PREPARE, Chennai. She currently works on HIV/AIDS, gender and primary health care and pesticide advocacy in Andhra Pradesh.
JUDE STEPHENS worked as Project Officer on HIV/AIDS-related work at PREPARE.

PREPARE is a national NGO working with tribals, fisherfolk and *dalits* since 1982 in the states of Tamil Nadu, Andhra Pradesh and Orissa. Its head office is in Chennai.

PREPARE,
4 Sathalvar Street,
Mugappair West, Chennai 600037.
Tel: 044-26244211
E-mail: prepare@vsnl.com

MEENA SESHU is General Secretary of SANGRAM, Sangli, Maharashtra State.

SANGRAM is an organisation that works with women in prostitution and sex work, rural women, young persons and adolescents to increase awareness about HIV/AIDS. SANGRAM believes that gender inequalities, stigma, discrimination and lack of treatment access for persons infected by HIV are fuelling the pandemic in India. Treatment and care of persons infected and affected by the HIV virus should be part of prevention efforts if the epidemic is to be checked in this country.

SANGRAM,
Aarohan,
Ghanshyam Nagar,
Madhav Nagar Road,
Sangli 416 416.
Tel: 0233-312 190
E-mail: san_meena@sancharnet.in

RADHIKA CHANDIRAMANI is the Director of TARSHI, New Delhi.

Based on the vision that all people have a right to sexual well-being and to a self-affirming and enjoyable sexuality, TARSHI works towards expanding sexual and reproductive choices in people's lives in an effort to enable them to enjoy lives of dignity, freedom from fear, infection, and reproductive and sexual health problems. TARSHI operates a telephone help line in Delhi since 1996. Informed by data and documentation on the concerns of people calling the help line, TARSHI has brought out publications on sexuality and related issues for diverse audiences such as young people, activists in the field of sexuality and professionals working in help line counselling related fields.

TARSHI (Talking About Reproductive and Sexual Health Issues),
11 Mathura Road, 1st Floor,
Jangpura B, New Delhi 110 014.
Phone: 011-2431 9070, 2431 9071
E-mail: rchandiramani@tarshi.com
Website: www.tarshi.org, www.sexualityinstitute.org, www.asiasrc.org

RADHIKA RAMASUBBAN is Director and BHANWAR RISHYASRINGA is Senior Fellow at the Centre for Social and Technological Change (CSTC), Mumbai.

Established in the early 1980s, the CSTC is an independent research group that is committed to generating and disseminating knowledge about economic and social development processes, particularly as they affect the poor in the country. The group's work has, over the years, focused on issues relating to food, energy, public health, drinking water, environmental sanitation and education.

Centre for Social and Technological Change,
Bandstand Apts, B.J. Road,
Bandra (W), Mumbai 400050.
Tel: 022-2641 8920
Fax: 022-2642 1969
E-mail: soctec@vsnl.com

SUNITI SOLOMON is the Director of the Y.R. Gaitonde Centre for AIDS Research and Education, Chennai.

YRG CARE provides prevention, care and support to people living with HIV and AIDS. It offers education on sexuality and HIV to adolescents and young adults; its continuum of care model caters to the prevention of HIV, reduces risks to HIV and other STIs, provides free access to confidential and anonymous counselling and testing services, runs an outpatient service for six days of the week, and a 24-hour, 21-bed in-patient ward. It also offers other support services to patients and their families. Besides prevention and care, YRG CARE is a medical and behavioural research centre and offers extensive training for clinicians, nurses, counsellors, educators and laboratory scientists.

Y.R. Gaitonde Centre for AIDS Research and Education (YRG CARE),
Voluntary Health Services,
Taramani, Chennai 600113.
Tel: 044-2254 2929
Fax: 044-2254 2939
Help line: 044-2254 2254
E-mail: info@yrgcare.org
Website: www.yrgcare.org

Introduction

RADHIKA RAMASUBBAN AND BHANWAR RISHYASRINGA

India is among the worst affected nations in the world in terms of the HIV/AIDS epidemic. Whether it is India or South Africa that has the largest number of HIV positive persons is putting too fine a point on what is clearly a very grim situation. The exact numbers may be disputed but there is no doubt in any quarters that they run into several millions. At last count by the National AIDS Control Organisation (NACO), there were over five million positive people in the country. This, too, could be just the proverbial tip of the iceberg, since the entire affected population can be counted only if people come forward for testing. It ought to be realised that even five million is the population of an average western European country. And, the numbers continue to grow, daily and invisibly, as the epidemic silently spreads among all sections of the population. The Indian epidemic, in fact, is believed to be one of the fastest growing HIV/AIDS epidemics in the world.

What is unique about HIV/AIDS in India is its combination of the medical nature of the disease (incurable), the main route of transmission (unprotected sex), the social exclusion spin-offs (stigma, discrimination), and the fact that the epidemic's spread in the country is fuelled by poverty, illiteracy and lack of education, unemployment, migration and the relative powerlessness of women vis-à-vis men. This is compounded by several cultural paradoxes. Strong cultural taboos prohibit open discussion about sex and sexuality, but allow for curiosity for sexual experimentation to slip through the cracks as long as it remains silent and without visible repercussions. Early, arranged and monogamous marriage is universally prescribed, where girls must be virgins and socialised into submissiveness within the four walls of the home but boys and men are permitted pre-marital and extra-marital experiences, and romantic love is celebrated in popular song and cinema. There are strict controls upon women's sexuality, but paid sex work is one of the few recourses open to poor, uneducated and unsupported women. The country has the world's highest rates of sexually transmitted infections, and one of the largest populations of sex workers, but the medical speciality that deals with the area of sexual health enjoys poor status, and sexual health education and counselling are conspicuously absent from the public domain.

Indian society is full of paradoxes. Its traditional music, poetry and sculpture celebrate romantic and erotic love, it gave the world the treatise of love and sex – the *Kamasutra* –, its great epics are full of stories of romantic attachments including outside of marriage and even accord a place – as the 'third sex' – to people of alternative sexualities. It is a diverse, open and fluid society in many respects. Yet, it is also driven by hierarchy and social exclusion as finely evolved social principles, making for a long tradition of discrimination relating to a range of social identities such as gender, caste, skin colour, disability, etc. It is a simple matter of extending these prejudices to a socially and medically complex disease such as HIV/AIDS.

HIV/AIDS highlights the failure of the country's economic and social development policies to secure economic stability and a healthy existence for all citizens, for it is those who are already socially and economically disadvantaged – predominantly poor people – who are most in danger of being sucked into the epidemic; and their numbers are huge. At the same time it holds a mirror, as never before, to some of the most intimate and problematic spaces in our cultural and personal environment. If HIV/AIDS were only the former, i.e., a developmental issue, it would have gone into a black box, just like our numerous other developmental problems. It is the latter, i.e., the deeply personal dimension, which has some potential to trigger off a process of social change.

What HIV/AIDS is doing is to challenge Indian society to turn itself inside-out: to focus on those sizeable sections of the population who were hitherto inconsequential, i.e., women and young people; and to bring those minorities who were hitherto invisible, 'untouchable' and unmentionable – prostitutes, men who have sex with men, *hijras* (transvestites), people disabled by the incurable affliction of HIV – out of the margins and into the centre. If the epidemic is to be controlled, the protection of these groups in terms of their human rights to health security, dignity, freedom of choice, and equality with other citizens is inseparable from the security of the rest of the society. What will tilt the scales in their favour and in the process set off eddies of change with repercussions for mainstream society, is if they develop a strong sense of agency. It is this process of empowerment that NGOs doing HIV/AIDS interventions are trying to assist in direct and indirect ways.

Non-governmental organisations (NGOs) – organisations that are voluntarily set up by individuals to perform self-help or socially useful roles – provide critical support to those vulnerable to the virus by helping them organise themselves, develop a sense of community and re-position themselves in relation to the rest of society. They work to prevent the spread of the virus through opening up channels for communication of protective information and awareness of rights among these groups. They make available treatment and care facilities to those who are already infected, in the process conferring on them social value, and advocate their cause among the mainstream medical profession. They work to bring about legal reform so that the civil rights of marginal groups and of affected and infected people are protected under the Constitution. They advocate the human rights of all vulnerable groups to be treated as citizens and not criminals, including the right to affordable medicines and treatment when they are sick. They seek to bring all these issues on to national agendas, and help stimulate regional and national networks in the common cause. They also work with similar groups based in other countries on common international platforms. The right to health security of all citizens has become a major advocacy issue, thanks to the stimulus provided by the HIV/AIDS epidemic.

This book showcases the work of six such NGOs. All have a track record of over a decade of dealing with an ever-expanding array of concerns in relation to the epidemic in India. What we have here are first person accounts by the individuals who built these institutions and whose names have become synonymous with the organisations that they set up. The reader can get a glimpse into the histories of their personal development, their growth paths as NGOs, and the mechanisms that they evolved to cope with new and unplanned developments in their chosen fields.

In this introductory essay, we first flesh out the main characteristics of HIV/AIDS as a disease and as a social issue, go on to briefly discuss the reasons that have propelled NGOs into the epidemic as key actors, followed by a short profile of the case studies themselves. The essay concludes with a discussion of the lessons that emerge from the case studies.

What is HIV/AIDS?

HIV/AIDS is a silent, symptomless infection caused by a virus – the human immunodeficiency virus (HIV) – that could enter the body during unprotected sexual encounters, through blood transfusions, infected needles or from mother to child. 'HIV positive' (or the oft-used word 'positive') denotes the presence in the infected person's body of the HIV virus; the production of specific antibodies is the immediate response of the body to any invasion by an outside pathogen – germ or infectious agent – and confirms that the body is harbouring that particular pathogen. Since HIV has no specific symptoms of its own until very late in the disease but only decreases the person's immunity, the person has no clue that he/she has contracted the infection until opportunistic infections start occurring. Only an 'HIV test' – ELISA test – and a further confirmatory test – Western Blot test – can identify the antibodies, and thus establish the 'HIV status' of a person, i.e., whether he/she is positive or not. Since the antibodies first appear in the blood only between six weeks and six months after the entry of the virus (an average of three months), any test that is conducted during this 'window period', i.e., when the 'seroconversion' is still taking place, will not show reliable results. Even if already done before, the tests must be repeated after the window period is over.

Because HIV/AIDS as a predominantly sexually transmitted and incurable disease tends to attract terrible stigma and discrimination against those who are infected, several international medical and human rights conventions have been formulated precisely in relation to this disease. These stipulate that every HIV test must be carried out with the full consent and knowledge of the person, accompanied by counselling and maintenance of confidentiality. Before the test, the person must receive 'pre-test counselling'. This includes complete information about the nature of the disease including factors in his/her own life that might have caused exposure to the infection, the nature of the test itself, and the implications if the test result is positive, negative or indeterminate. The person is then offered the choice of undergoing the test; this is known as 'informed consent'. If the person tests positive, he/she must mandatorily be offered 'post-test counselling' that maintains the 'confidentiality' of the person's positive status. Post-test counselling is meant to help the person come to terms with the diagnosis, learn how to make responsible changes in lifestyle and how to take care of himself/herself, particularly in terms of nutrition and treatment for opportunistic infections.

The uniqueness of the HIV virus is that it attacks the immune system itself, making the body steadily incapable of fighting common infections. In course of time the person becomes 'immuno-deficient' and susceptible to what are called 'opportunistic infections', well known communicable illnesses such as tuberculosis, bacterial pneumonia, herpes zoster, mouth ulcers, skin diseases, etc., which take on particularly stubborn form in positive patients and require aggressive treatment. These infections are curable if attended to promptly and by doctors skilled in treating these infections in HIV positive patients ('HIV management'). Prompt treatment combined with good nutrition, regular exercise and a positive mental outlook can keep an HIV positive person looking and feeling normal and healthy and leading an active and useful life just like anyone else. However, the person continues to remain highly infectious and can transmit the virus, through sexual intercourse where condoms are not used, or if he/she donates blood that goes untested, or shares unsterilised needles if he/she is an intravenous drug user or has a child if the person is a pregnant woman.

At this point, a positive person has the option to go in for a set of complex tests, i.e., absolute CD4/CD8 count and its percentage and ratio. The CD4 cell count in the blood – a type of white blood cells – establishes the level of immunity, since CD4 counts start decreasing as the infection progresses. When the CD4 count goes below 200, the person is a definite candidate for beginning combination 'anti-retroviral therapy' (ART). Combination ART consists of three anti-retroviral drugs mixed together to prevent drug resistance, that brings down the viral load, boosts the immune system and delays further damage to it, and holds out the real possibility of improving the quality of life and longevity of those already infected. However, since the disease itself is incurable, ART is a life-long treatment. Essentially, it enables the patient to manage the disease just as any other incurable and chronic degenerative diseases such as diabetes or Alzheimer's disease. ART, however, is not a substitute to continuing with condom use, as the person can continue to transmit the virus during unprotected intercourse.

ART has several built-in drawbacks. It is expensive, complicated to administer, has several side effects, and requires regular monitoring for CD4 counts, viral load and drug resistance. Regular visits to and counselling by the treating physician, and emotional support from family or friends are essential accompanying factors. Failure to be meticulous in following the dosage schedule, either because of irregular supply or haphazard intake, can lead to drug resistance in the patient. If the person becomes complacent that he/she is being protected by the drugs – something that can happen easily in the case of all life-long treatments – and lapses into unprotected sex, it could result in the spread of drug-resistant HIV. All these drawbacks make ART a difficult option for those who are disadvantaged in terms of income, education, social/psychological support and self-discipline. But for those who can afford it and follow it with meticulous precision, ART can offer tremendous advantages.

Even without ART, an HIV positive person who is economically and socially secure may expect to remain reasonably healthy for many years. At some point, when the body's immune system breaks down beyond repair and opportunistic illnesses become more frequent, chronic and damaging, the person moves into the more acute and terminal form of the disease known as 'AIDS'. Once this occurs, the person becomes prey to a whole host of persistent illnesses such as Cytomegalovirus (CMV), Pneumocystis carinii Pneumonia (PCP), and various cancers some of which are peculiar to the AIDS condition and severe loss of body weight leading to death.

Through all these stages from HIV through AIDS, the person can transmit the virus to others only through exchange of body fluids such as semen, vaginal secretions, blood/blood products or breast milk. HIV/AIDS is, thus, not a randomly acquired infection, but travels only along these definite routes. In India, 85 per cent of infections are transmitted through sex. Touch, saliva, sweat, air, mosquitoes or shared common spaces such as homes, offices, swimming pools, or toilets do not constitute transmission routes. Nor can the HIV virus survive outside of the body. Despite these scientifically established facts, several misconceptions abound regarding HIV transmission, and fuel the terrible stigma and discrimination surrounding this disease. It is wrong to believe that one can recognise an HIV positive person by his/her appearance and therefore avoid them. Or that touching a positive person, or breathing the same air, or sitting and eating together could cause transmission to take place.

HIV/AIDS almost always occurs in limited, known and well-defined situations, i.e., sex with partners whose own sexual history has involved multiple partners, presence of untreated sexually transmitted infections in one or both partners, presence of reproductive tract inflammations or infections among women partners, use of infected needles, transfusion of infected blood, and unsafe hospital practices. Of these, multiple sexual partners and a high incidence of sexually transmitted infections constitute the most common situation. In India, there are a few groups that tend most to have multiple sexual partners (such as sex workers, migrant workers, truck drivers and men who have sex with men). But these groups are not watertight compartments. They have active linkages with the mainstream society resulting in much sexual mixing, as we will describe later.

Finally, HIV/AIDS can be prevented through self-conscious knowledge and the power of individual and collective action, i.e., correct and consistent use of condoms, prompt treatment of sexually transmitted infections and reproductive tract infections, using blood that has tested safe and adhering to 'universal precautions' (ensuring the sterility of all invasive medical instruments including injection needles [and needles of drug users], consistent use of protective clothing in hospitals where necessary and careful disposal of wastes contaminated by pus, blood and other bodily secretions). Of these, condom use has the potential of widest impact, since sexual intercourse is the commonest behaviour, and the sexually active population constitutes more than 50 per cent of the already huge Indian population.

In India, condom use is abysmally low. The Indian family planning programme initially promoted it as a family planning method – Nirodh – but the decision to concentrate all efforts on sterilising women rather than on persuading men to also share responsibility of contraception led to condoms even as a contraceptive method fading into insignificance. To revive it now in the context of HIV, as a prevention method against sexually transmitted disease and to bring men back into the picture, is an uphill task.

Social aspects of HIV/AIDS

The problem arises when individuals are not able to acquire the protective knowledge, or exercise autonomous preventive action, due to overpowering 'social contexts of risks' which trap them and over which they have little or no control. The most potent of these social contexts are oppressive frameworks of sexuality, compounded by poverty and gender inequalities. Unsafe health care environments that do not observe universal precautions, too, are contexts of risk. Hence, although theoretically everybody in society is at risk of contracting HIV infection, the scales are tilted against those who are disadvantageously placed in relation to any or all of the above social contexts.

Gender inequality and culturally moulded notions of what it is to be a 'man-as-a-sexual-being' and men's 'legitimate' sexual expectations from wives, result in women's unquestioning subordination to men's sexual desires, and rob women of autonomy in relation to their own bodies. This may be more acutely manifested in conditions of dire poverty, where sexual dominance over wives (often accompanied by violence) may be used by men as a compensatory mechanism to cope with their own economic fragility, aided by alcohol and other forms of substance abuse.

Social double standards permit boys and men lax sexual norms but expect 'innocence' and ignorance about sex from girls. The taboos on access to correct sexuality-related information mean that boys and girls and even adult men and women labour under many misconceptions, fears and doubts relating to their own sexuality and sexual health. Men and boys are particularly affected by fears and doubts regarding sexual performance, and tend to remain preoccupied with confirming their abilities in this regard, often through visits to commercial sex workers. Such sexual behaviours could lead to men falling prey to sexually transmitted infections and then passing them on to their wives. Due to the nature of women's biology, sexually transmitted infections move much more effectively from men to women than vice versa. Adolescent and young women are in even greater danger of such infections due to the physiological immaturity of the cervix and genital tract, which make the entry of the HIV virus into the body even easier. The young age at which women in India marry and that their sex life actively begins soon thereafter, puts them at great risk if their husbands have engaged in risky pre-marital sex. Marriage is fast emerging as the greatest risk factor for women in India in the context of HIV/AIDS. Since men seeking paid sex and fearing HIV infection are demanding virgins and very young girls, criminal syndicates trafficking in women are bringing ever-younger girls into prostitution. Scientific studies show that rates of HIV infection are higher among young girls and women than among older women. Worst affected by cultural taboos and social double standards are those whose sexuality does not even conform to the dominant gender norms of heterosexuality. These are the minority groups of people with alternative sexualities – notably homosexuals, also known as men who have sex with men –, who have to resort to great secrecy in matters to do with their own personal identity.

Poverty acts to worsen the effects of the above social and cultural influences. Widespread poverty keeps people from school and leaves them too illiterate to correctly absorb and retain protective health information that they encounter in random public places, like pamphlets or hoardings or TV advertisements. Poverty forces men to migrate in search of work and endure long periods of separation from their wives. This makes them vulnerable to seeking out paid sex. They may also resort to anal sex with other men or boys as alternatives in such situations (seen as release of sexual energy or heat from the body, and not 'real sex'); this may happen more frequently in situations where older men and young boys are thrown together. Anal sex is the most efficient among the sexual routes, but condoms are almost never used in these encounters. These men may contract sexually transmitted infections including HIV, from each other or from commercial sex workers, which they then transmit to others in the chain including their wives.

When poverty combines with the fact of being a woman – in a society where girl children are at a discount – the consequences could become even worse. When women test positive – as when they go to health centres for pregnancy tests – they may be castigated by their families as immoral and thrown out of the house. When their babies are born HIV positive and die, they are seen as total failures in their role as mothers. And when the positive husband dies, they may be thrown out of the home or denied a share in his property. Without education or skills, women who become destitute and/or deserted by their husbands may be forced into prostitution to purchase economic security. The chain of HIV transmission and human tragedy could thus go on and on.

Certain groups in society have an even greater vulnerability to the virus than those in the conditions described above. Labelled 'high risk groups', these are women in prostitution, men who have sex with men, truck drivers and migrant workers. What unites them is their sexual behaviour: multiple sex partners, failure to use condoms, susceptibility to sexually transmitted infections, and delays in seeking sexual health care due to fears of discrimination, particularly among those who practise anal sex. Almost all of them are also married, including the men who have sex with men, since marriage is virtually universal – a family duty, a social obligation – in Indian society. And women in prostitution, too, almost always have regular lovers or husband-like figures to whom they are devoted as if in a marital relationship. Within these relationships, again, as within marriage, condoms are never used. The distinctive nature of the Indian epidemic is that the sexual networks through which HIV transmission is taking place in the society are fairly intermeshed and widespread as described here, and not confined only to small 'high risk' groups.

Why NGOs?

Stemming the tide of the HIV/AIDS epidemic in the country requires action on the fronts opened up by all of the above cultural, social and economic contexts.

One action is political will on the part of the government to implement progressive social and economic development policies that start making visible impact on some of these 'contexts of risk' such as poverty, unemployment, illiteracy and migration. Fostering a progressive and efficient policy environment for HIV/AIDS control programmes is another important arena of responsibility of the government. A crucial aspect of this is to raise the profile of anti-HIV/AIDS efforts, to forge links between the objectives and work of the National AIDS Control Organisation (NACO) – the apex body for AIDS control efforts in the country – and the other arms of the government, and between HIV/AIDS control programmes and public health programmes. At present, even within the government, AIDS control remains outside the mainstream with the NACO working in isolation.

A second action is direct intervention at the level of local communities, particularly those that are at greatest risk, to prevent the further spread of infection, and to safeguard the human rights to dignity, economic security and quality medical treatment of those who are already affected. Such intervention efforts need to be deliberately planned, sensitively designed and implemented, and long term in nature. Non-governmental organisations (NGOs) are the main intervention agencies in this regard.

A third action is citizens' commitment to what one might describe as a 'common social project' with respect to HIV/AIDS. The features of such a project should be a higher level of public understanding and debate about health and human rights for all, and a more compassionate, liberal and human rights-sensitive social environment which accords equality to vulnerable groups with the rest of society, free of discrimination and stigma. For this to happen, it is very important for all citizens – and that includes lawyers, judges, doctors, entrepreneurs, police, teachers, students, factory and informal sector workers, peasants, home-makers, and indeed everybody – to seek out and acquire basic information about HIV and through their attitudes, help positive people integrate into the rest of society, and reduce the unnecessary burden of stigma carried by them. Also, it is only when HIV/AIDS becomes everybody's business and concern that there will emerge the necessary public pressure for more effective policies for its control. This requires going beyond relying solely on the general media for information, where reporting is most often superficial and often sensational.

Three factors make NGOs important in the context of HIV/AIDS in India.

The sensitive nature of the social risks and the sexual routes of transmission of the HIV virus, described earlier, require interventions that assure confidentiality and anonymity to those who access these services. They need to be fine-tuned to local situations, and small enough in scale to permit learning, flexibility and mid-course corrections. Sexuality is one of the most personal and intimate areas of people's lives, an area that they would not wish to talk about within a formal, impersonal or hierarchical environment, i.e., one that lacks in confidentiality. Any hint of being exposed, judged in negative ways, slighted, or rejected would be enough to restrain them from talking about anything that troubles them with regard to their sexuality or sexual health. Also, in Indian society, there are such strong overtones of 'immorality' that are directed at anyone who speaks about sexual problems with regard to themselves, that people would prefer to remain silent rather than become the butt of ridicule or condemnation. In such a situation, it is only within highly confidential spaces where anonymity and/or confidentiality is assured that people, whose life circumstances or sexual behaviour put them at risk of HIV infection, would be willing to open up to seek knowledge, advice or help. NGOs working in the HIV/AIDS field – as different from large impersonal bureaucracies, government-run institutions, or mass media – offer such 'safe' spaces. They tend to be small-scale organisations that are stably based in local communities and enjoy the trust and confidence of the members of these communities.

Secondly, the unprecedented stigma and discrimination levelled by society at large against those affected by the disease –

paralleled only by the stigma reserved for leprosy patients in an earlier era –, require interventions with a heavy counselling component, i.e., repeated face-to-face confidential and respectful interaction between skilled counsellors and those affected by the stigma, that can help people cope with these assaults and gradually become empowered to re-approach their lives with a new sense of purpose. Ostracism, desperation and depression can lead to more irresponsible behaviour (such as visiting sex workers without using a condom) or even to suicide. For those who are already vulnerable to the disease due to their sexuality such as women in prostitution, men who have sex with men, or persons of alternative sexualities, the hostile and stigma-ridden social climate has only worsened with HIV/AIDS, sometimes resulting in hate crimes. To reach them in the first place and persuade them to change their behaviour and life circumstances with a view to ensure their own safety, requires intensive and sustained interaction, advocacy, and the provision of facilities for testing, treatment and rehabilitation. Only those with high levels of commitment to working for less privileged and stigmatised groups, and willing to 'soil their hands' (and reputations) would be willing to make an entry. Such interventions are necessarily exploratory in nature; they expand gradually in response to demands from and participation by the populations being served. None of these conditions is compatible with what we know of the government's style of functioning. Large government-driven programmes run by faceless bureaucracies may do well in vaccination campaigns as in the case of small pox vaccination and revaccination in the 1960s or pulse polio in the 1990s, but fail when sensitivity to individual situations and flexibility are called for. The result is that today in the HIV/AIDS sector, a wide range of NGOs bears a heavy burden of carrying prevention, treatment and care, and advocacy and legal aid services to vulnerable groups and people. These NGOs operate in far-flung corners of the country.

Finally, since the earliest days of the epidemic in India, NGOs have been the principal firefighters, responding to real and immediate issues. And these issues have been several: arrests and indefinite imprisonment of positive persons; forced deportations of sex workers by the governments of the states where they live to their states of origin; dismissal of employees from jobs upon their testing positive; and women and their children being thrown out by their husbands' families when found positive. The reasons are historical. For several years after HIV surfaced in India, society in general and the government in particular were in a state of denial about the possibility that HIV/AIDS could ever become a serious problem in India. The generally held belief was that AIDS was a foreign and culturally alien – 'immoral' – disease that could not be indigenous to a society that sanctioned only heterosexuality and monogamous arranged marriages, upheld women as mothers and worshipped them as goddesses. 'Indian culture' was believed to be an impregnable bulwark against any sexually transmitted infection. Since the international scientific literature had identified high rates of partner change as the cause of spread of the HIV virus, and since sex workers by virtue of their occupation are most prone to a large number of partners, the government believed that compulsorily testing sex workers, arresting and isolating those found infected, and generally keeping controls on visiting foreigners – unprotected as they were by Indian culture –, were sufficient measures. Similar treatment was meted out to others who showed up as positive for the virus. During those long years of denial, the only constructive response to the threat of spread of HIV infection came from civil society – generally professionals such as medical researchers, doctors, social workers, lawyers –, idealistic persons willing to intervene in an uncharted and stigmatised terrain. As their understanding of the disease and its manifold social ramifications grew, these NGOs saw the need for flexible organisational structures within which they could learn and innovate as they went along. It is under this compulsion that many of the earliest HIV/AIDS non-governmental organisations were born and took shape.

NGOs in HIV/AIDS are an inseparable part of the larger national NGO sector, which is the most visible face of civil society activism in India today. Many NGOs see their role as one of bringing to the development process a combination of professionalism and service to those in greatest need, that they see missing from the top-down delivery of development programmes by government agencies. India has witnessed a steady burgeoning of the NGO sector. The experience of the Emergency – the first ever abrogation of democratic rights in independent India –, the disillusionment with government-administered development programmes that did not seem to be making a dent on mass poverty, the revival of the Gandhian concern for rural development and service to the poorest of the poor, particularly in the countryside, and the ideal of harnessing professional expertise to concerns of equity, led to the emergence of a vigorous voluntary sector in the social landscape beginning from the late 1970s. Many of these 'voluntary groups' as they were known then were led by doctors and engineers, who also saw their roles as taking modern science and technology to the masses. Today, the Indian NGO sector has become huge – one of the largest in the world – and is accorded importance as one among the three most important sectors in the country along with the government and the private sector.

NGOs are aware that individually they are small oases in a sea of problems, and while their independent stance gives them the satisfaction of being able to follow their own paths, they have few illusions that they can bring about large-scale transformation. Those with dynamic leadership see themselves as demonstrating the 'art of the possible', innovating models for intervening and changing society, that can be emulated by other NGOs and scaled up by larger agencies such as the government. Their advocacy efforts – trying to change the way society looks at the particular problem and the way those affected by it view themselves – are also central to the complex of roles that they see for themselves as change agents. Nor are they committed to operating in isolation. With globalisation, NGOs find it possible to be part of international information-sharing networks and funding arrangements. They also look to network with others like themselves within the country for advocacy around their common causes. They willingly collaborate with the government on planning and decision-making committees.

The alliances between NGOs and their non-NGO partners, however, may not always be easy and non-controversial. The NGOs in this book, for example, are all grounded in a human rights approach to HIV/AIDS that puts the individual at the centre and upholds the principles of social justice, equity and non-discrimination. The Government of India, too, is a signatory to international conventions that commit it to secure the health of its citizens in terms of 'rights' rather than simply 'needs'. By doing so, the government accepts accountability for making available health provisions and services, and making health care environments safe, without excuses of financial constraints or discriminatory priorities. However, other policies of the government may go against this commitment. The most recent and ongoing controversy relates to the amendments to the Patent Act of 1970 that has been recently passed by the Indian Parliament. NGOs fear that the amended Act will cause drug prices in the country to shoot up, putting treatment for ill health, including HIV/AIDS-related illness, even more out of the reach of the country's poor.

It is notable that in the Indian HIV/AIDS sector, funds for interventions come overwhelmingly from international donor agencies such as the World Bank and the UN system, bilateral agencies such as the British government's Department for International Development (DFID), and private foundations such as the Ford Foundation in the early days, and more recently the Bill and Melinda Gates Foundation and Richard Gere Foundation. Given the initial state of denial in India, and having seen HIV/AIDS at close quarters in their own countries and witnessed how combined efforts of government, industry and civil society can make for successful policies for control of the epidemic, these donors believe that their support for Indian efforts might make a difference to the direction of the epidemic in India and prevent the repetition of the African experience where large parts of that continent have been devastated by HIV/AIDS.

Almost all funds are earmarked for prevention work, i.e., condom distribution, HIV/AIDS awareness raising, and treatment of sexually transmitted infections. NGOs whose work involves providing treatment and care services find themselves cash strapped, with virtually no sources to turn to. Nearly seventeen years into the epidemic and with the stepping up of intervention efforts, more and more people are testing positive, and positive people who had hitherto been relatively invisible are now getting sicker and are approaching the health services as patients. But mainstream services are still reluctant to admit positive persons as in-patients, while outpatients continue to face discrimination and/or exorbitant fees by doctors and medical staff who are most often unskilled in treating HIV patients. There are any numbers of quacks who offer AIDS cures, and patients and their families crowd to them but soon find themselves financially ruined. After doing their rounds of quacks and mainstream doctors, these patients – by then often having sold off their property and burdened by mounting debts – eventually arrive at the doors of specialised services in the NGO sector. Here they are treated with compassion and dignity, nursed back to a semblance of health, and their families are taught how to care for them once they are back home, all at a nominal cost. The NGOs who offer such holistic care are few in number and find themselves overstretched financially, besides the frustration of having to treat patients who are in an advanced stage of sickness.

It is imperative for international donors and government policy makers to see prevention and care as inseparably linked, since educating people about prevention and the importance of testing is tantamount to prompting them to seek health care from services which continue to reject them. Three of the NGOs in this book who started off as advocates for prevention found themselves having to expand into testing, treatment and care since members of the public who were responding to their educational efforts had nowhere else to go for good quality and respectful care.

The HIV/AIDS epidemic in the Western countries has also spawned vocal 'patient groups' that have consistently lobbied their governments for more money for research into HIV vaccines and drugs, raised issues for public debate on laws impinging on vulnerable groups, and set norms for the general involvement of the public in issues relating to human rights and individual and social responsibility. This has prompted many foreign donors and UN agencies working in India to stipulate that HIV positive people (known as 'People Living with HIV/AIDS' [PLWHA]) be represented in national and regional committees that frame policies and set priorities for intervention. One of the outcomes of this prescription is that such PLWHA groups have come into existence in many states in the country. These are still fledgeling organisations, consisting of persons hailing from already socially disadvantaged groups – since positive people who are well off would prefer to buy expensive anti-retroviral treatment and keep their identity secret rather than make common cause with poor, stigmatised groups – who require to develop the skills needed to play the roles taken on by their counterparts in other countries. It is, nevertheless, a unique phenomenon, since such patient groups do not exist in the case of any other communicable disease in the country such as TB or leprosy. One of the advocacy platforms adopted by these groups is for affordable health care for HIV positive people. The success of their efforts would be contingent on their evolution into powerful advocates for their cause. But they are not alone. A coalition of NGOs in the country spearheaded by one of the NGOs in this book has been waging a struggle since 2001 – the Affordable Medicines and Treatment Campaign – to convince the Government of India that its proposed amendments to its Patent Act of 1970 militate against the government's own avowed commitment to the human right to health of its citizens.

A major new factor in the globalisation of the AIDS discourse is the recent demonstration by Indian pharmaceutical firms of the capability to produce and internationally market vastly cheaper (generic) and more accessibly formulated – a single three dose combination which reduces the number of pills to be consumed per day – anti-retroviral drugs than the patented drugs available in developed country markets. In doing so, these firms were exploiting the Indian patent policies of the pre-WTO era, i.e., patents on processes but not on products. By innovating with the basic processes, these generic firms were able to come up with the new generation of ARV drugs. The low cost of the drugs has led to their being exported to other developing countries such as Brazil, Thailand and South Africa whose governments are committed to providing free/affordable ART to their citizens. This post-2000 development also provided a fillip to the agenda of patient groups in the rich countries, in solidarity with patient groups in developing countries, for easier access to more affordable drugs for all. Cheaper AIDS drugs also have the potential to revolutionise HIV/AIDS care in the long run by removing the stigma that attaches to a disease that is equated with being a death sentence.

It is this chain of revolutionary developments that the amendments to the Patent Act, passed by the Indian Parliament recently, has set back. Under the new amendments, patent protection will be extended to both processes and products and any new use of known drugs, thus assuring the indefinite extension of the market monopoly of developed country pharmaceutical manufacturers with the attendant high prices. This will impact on all essential and life-saving drugs, in addition to ARVs.

The task of working at the grassroots in the flexible and sensitive manner described earlier, responding to local challenges each demanding its own unique response, and taking up advocacy at the national level, is a difficult undertaking. In the HIV/AIDS sector, the 'soft' nature of the interventions – empowering women and men and youth to take responsibility in relation to their sexuality, sexual relations and sexual health, and struggling to get government to focus on people's health rights – and the extended time frame that they require to be implemented over, makes them difficult to assess in terms of concrete outcomes. A few studies have investigated the effectiveness of interventions among homogenous and organised communities. The best known example is that of the sex workers in Sonagachi in Kolkata, led by their own organisation – the Durbar Mahila Samanwaya Committee – where a successful intervention programme was able to record an increase in condom use and decrease in sexually transmitted diseases and HIV, a growing self awareness as a community with common concerns, and a greater desire to integrate themselves into the Indian mainstream as equal citizens.

Case studies

The case studies in the book include YRG CARE and PREPARE in Chennai, Naz Foundation (India) Trust and TARSHI in Delhi, SANGRAM in Sangli district of Maharashtra, and the Lawyers Collective in Mumbai, Delhi and Bangalore.

The manner in which a medical scientist's early initiative evolved and resulted in the formation of YRG CARE – an organisation that has become a synonym for high quality, humane and affordable care and a model worthy of replication – offers several interesting insights into the birth and evolution of an HIV/AIDS non-government organisation. This was the first multifaceted and constructive response to the epidemic in the state of Tamil Nadu, one of the highest prevalence states in the country. Such an early entry into the field, persistence after the initial entry, self-definition as a learning organisation with relation to the medical and social ramifications of the disease, willingness to expand into new and unknown directions and build a wide range of partnerships, and engagement with the public from the very start, all mark it as a pioneer. It is probably significant in the Indian context that this initiative came from within the formal professional medical structure, a structure which even today is the most stubborn bastion of stigma directed against positive persons. Two activities of YRG CARE are unique to it within the historical context in which they were launched, that may be traced to this medical-professional identity. Since its earliest days it has been doing adolescent sexuality education, both within educational institutions and within community-based structures. YRG CARE was able to use the authoritative and non-subversive image that medical professionals in the country enjoy to gain the confidence of school principals and teachers and community opinion leaders in launching this initiative. Their predominantly medical background was also a facilitating factor in the group's entry into the arena of treatment and care. Not only were they able to perceive early in the epidemic the snowballing effect of offering the continuum of public education, counselling and testing, leading to support and treatment, they were also professionally equipped to offer this treatment and care. A very important aspect of its professional identity that YRG CARE has consistently and zealously guarded is its continuing engagement with clinical research. This is surely a factor that keeps taut the creative tension of the organisation's growth path. For YRG CARE, the iterative learning afforded by the interaction with the global scientific community, while being firmly grounded in the local reality of delivering treatment and working for prevention in the southern Indian region, is central to its ability to sustain itself intellectually. That its research collaborations also yield it valuable funds that it channels into drugs and medicines for its patients, and buying newer generations of testing equipment, is a bonus.

PREPARE's experience is that of a developmental NGO working among the poorest communities, that unexpectedly found itself having to respond to the problem of HIV/AIDS in its project area. This case study brings to the fore the introspections an NGO may have to go through before getting involved in the sensitive issues that HIV/AIDS work involves. PREPARE members asked themselves whether they were sufficiently prepared in terms of their own attitudes and deep-rooted reservations regarding linkages of HIV/AIDS with sexuality issues. Leadership by practice was an important factor here in helping younger members of the team to confront their own prejudices, and learn to respect the freedom of others to choose their own sexual behaviour and sexual orientation. The particular intervention reported here – prevention education and treatment for sexually transmitted and reproductive tract infections among industrial workers, many of them migrants and a large proportion of them women – involved organisational learning and coming up with innovations in a virgin field. The intervention involved experimenting with a series of strategies and choices: how to build mutually non-conflicting partnerships with managements, workers and trade unions; how to work with different gender and age groups within the factory environment; how to design education programmes that could be effectively delivered within the time spaces permitted by the managements; how to combine the factory level interventions with interventions in workers' housing colonies; how to co-opt local hospitals for treatment and care, and local social hubs as 'change agents' for prevention education; and how to extend prevention education to the spouses of vulnerable migrant workers living in their native villages.

TARSHI is a telephone help line service that offers sexuality-related information. It also produces sexuality-related materials for diverse audiences. Its focus is on young people and their sexuality, and its objective is to free them from the shackles of misconceptions, fears, violence and infections that they carry due to lack of accurate and user-friendly information about sexuality, and to promote the understanding of sexuality as a positive force for physical and mental well-being. The help line uses every opportunity afforded by callers to convey information about safe sex and HIV infection and prevention. The case study documents the extent of ignorance about sex and anatomy and the most elementary bodily processes among young people, and highlights the huge demand for sexuality education that is out there in the society, as revealed by the number and nature of questions callers put to the help line. It is noteworthy that the maximum calls even in a big metropolis are from boys and men; girls and women continue to be very inhibited about finding out more about their bodies. It is a story of the sensitive and exacting nature of a sexuality-related help line, the dilemmas posed by the help line's commitment to confidentiality and anonymity particularly when callers demonstrate severe mental disturbance, depression or the threat/fear of impending violence, the kind of attributes that are required for counsellors on the job, the importance of continuous training and motivation of counsellors, and the high rate of burnout among them.

The basic position of SANGRAM that works among women in prostitution is that women in prostitution are as much in need of protection as the rest of mainstream society. Their lives and health are valuable in their own right. Women in prostitution have relative control over some aspects of their lives – sexuality, reproduction, relationships – as compared with non-prostitute women, and they do not always see themselves as victims. They are willing to be proactive in matters impinging on their lives rather than cower before others for protection. The challenge is how to empower them to protect themselves; this is SANGRAM's mission. The story is about a trained social worker's decision to work among women from the *devadasi* community in a red light area in Maharashtra – one of the highest HIV prevalence states in the country –, her experience of establishing rapport with the women, the setbacks that she encounters in gaining their confidence and trust and the manner in which she tries to get around the obstacles, the experiments in capacity building, leading finally to the establishment of a collective of women in prostitution. Today, these women are proud of their identity as card-holding members of the collective. The chapter provides insights into the process of partnering with other agencies, particularly the vicissitudes of building partnerships with the government; details the strategies employed to extend the work of HIV/AIDS prevention into the mainstream society among married household women, adolescent youth, school and college students, all of which groups are closely linked to the women in prostitution through the 'bridging behaviours' of men and boys; and documents the process of introspection and self-evaluation of this overall growth path.

Naz Foundation (India) Trust offers prevention and care services under the umbrella of its overarching principle that HIV/AIDS is first and foremost a human rights issue. Naz accordingly works among a range of social groups – health care professionals, college students, women's groups – to raise awareness about HIV and the rights of people who are vulnerable to and infected with the virus. Much of the chapter is devoted to Naz's exploration of prevention and care strategies appropriate to men who have sex with men (MSM), where it is a pioneer in the country. It is a story of identifying and bringing MSM into the open, of balancing the tension between advocacy and service provision, and of confronting the ever-present dilemma of client confidentiality and the challenges involved in helping individuals along the path of empowerment and decision-making. It also recounts how one thing led to another and Naz found itself taking on the production of condoms suited to MSM sexual activity. Finally, it is a story of networking, and of mobilising representatives of gay rights, women's rights, child rights, health and human rights organisations to decriminalise the status of MSM in the Indian legal system.

The Lawyers Collective HIV/AIDS Unit has been the pioneering organisation in the country in relation to formulating approaches to the legal protection of those affected by the virus. Against the background of the crucial role played by public interest litigations in highlighting major contentious social issues, their successes and failures, the chapter emphasises the need for debate, discussion and advocacy outside of the courts for the realisation of the full potential of legal remedies for the benefit of the poor. It documents the story of the struggle to frame legal instruments for the employment security of HIV positive persons, for the protection of their right to consent, confidentiality and freedom from discrimination in the matters of testing, marriage, employment, health care, education and exposure in the media. It is a story of a lawyer's movement from personal involvement to institution building and capacity development, of the expansion into different geographical regions, of moving the legal agenda forward through the instrument of polemical journal articles for the public and advocacy workshops for a whole range of stakeholders. It discusses how the institution building process requires constant talent hunting, the ability to sustain young lawyers within an NGO framework against the lure of more lucrative opportunities outside, coming to terms with the simultaneously liberating and sullying effects of money within development activities, and the development of grassroots capabilities. The principal lesson is that it is not the success or failure of legal remedies alone that is critical; collective organisation and self-generated advocacy around legal issues can become a powerful source of sustenance for vulnerable groups.

Lessons

The case studies suggest that NGOs see themselves as serious partners of the government in tackling the HIV/AIDS epidemic in the country. All the NGOs in the book have eagerly responded to the government's call for NGO participation in the National AIDS Control Programme, whether it involves distributing condoms at the grassroots as in the case of SANGRAM and its sister collective of sex workers VAMP, or serving on technical and scientific advisory committees in the manner of YRG CARE and the Naz Foundation, or spearheading a nation-wide consultative process around framing a new legislation for the HIV/AIDS epidemic as in the case of the Lawyers Collective.

In many parts of the country, however, particularly as one moves closer to the ground at the district and sub-district levels, the government's expectation from NGOs is that they should be performing their roles as submissive service providers and as sub-contractors in government projects, acquiescing to a patron-client relationship with the district bureaucracy rather than as partners in a national cause. NGOs, on the other hand, see themselves as agents of change, as taking responsibility for joint ownership of government programmes, and bring a missionary zeal to their work. In fact, it is their holistic approach – their conceptual and ideological links with the larger canvas – and their sense of mission that give them the vibrancy that marks them out from routine bureaucratic approaches. All of these attributes, however, tend to be resented by the bureaucratic and the political elites at the local level, who continue to subscribe to feudal symbols of prestige, power and hierarchy.

Nor do their government partners at the local level always appreciate the gender sensitivity that characterises NGO interventions. The persecution of SANGRAM and VAMP activists by the local police and elected representatives was in keeping with patriarchal double standards that deny women in prostitution civil rights, but are liberal in their dispensation to the male clients of prostitutes. PREPARE recognised the constraints on married women workers of having to combine factory labour with domestic responsibilities and commuting, leaving them with no time to attend the NGO's educational sessions held after factory hours; the NGO accordingly modified its intervention strategy in order to include the women. A universal feature of treatment seeking behaviour across the country as highlighted by numerous research studies is that men access clinic services more than do women, given gender inequalities in access to household funds, freedom of movement outside the house especially to distant medical facilities, or household support for adult members suffering ill health. The Naz Foundation's Care Home, for example, explicitly recognises this and encourages very sick positive women to get admitted as in-patients for up to a month at a time so they can receive treatment and get the rest that they would not otherwise in their busy households, where women are expected to uncomplainingly shoulder the entire burden of housework.

Given that 'mainstreaming' is the current buzzword, how would NGOs collaborating on government programmes ensure that their own initiative and work style are not cramped? Or that women – whose cause they particularly espouse – get their due? How would these sensitive components be mainstreamed? This raises several questions for NGOs: how much should NGOs be willing to compromise in order to participate in government programmes? Should NGOs at all become part of government programmes? Should they concentrate on scaling themselves up to acquire wider impact? Or should they continue to remain small and integrated with their own ideals?

NGOs collaborating with the government also find themselves having to simultaneously play the role of watchdogs, particularly at the national level. This takes the form of advocacy/public protests, to highlight the iniquitous nature of government policies or human rights violations that contradict the government's own professed commitments to the welfare of its citizens, or that go against the spirit and letter of international covenants that the government is a signatory to. The actions by SANGRAM/VAMP and NAZ as part of their respective national networks for decriminalisation of sex work and consensual same sex activity, respectively, and of the Affordable Medicines and

Treatment Campaign of which the Lawyers Collective is a part, are cases in point.

Admittedly, the human right to health and to affordable treatment for all has only been obliquely recognised by the Indian State. This is evident from the low level of political, financial and administrative commitment to public health, resulting in the appalling state of preventive and curative health services in the country's public sector. Even the poorest sections of society perceive the public services as inadequate and of poor quality, and resort to expensive private providers when in distress. However, what has catapulted HIV/AIDS as a disease into the rights discourse in an unprecedented way – and, thereby, actually given a new fillip to the issue of health as a human right as espoused by NGOs – are two interrelated factors.

One is the right to knowledge. This arises from the fact that HIV/AIDS is only in part a disease; it is even more a cultural, social, economic and developmental problem. Social taboos on gaining accurate knowledge about sexuality and sexual health, lax sexual norms for men in such an environment of lack of information and misinformation, cultural values that place women at a disadvantage in relation to men and in terms of access to knowledge about their own bodies and about the world outside, poverty, unemployment and migration are some of the factors that fuel individual sexual behaviours that make people vulnerable to HIV/AIDS. Further, HIV/AIDS is a fatal incurable disease, and prevention is the only known method of avoiding it. Therefore, a crucial element is the individual's right to know about prevention: how to avoid acquiring the infection and, if infected, how to prevent spreading it. HIV focuses the spotlight on this right to knowledge as never before. In a most fundamental sense, the right to know is embedded in the right to life itself.

The other factor to the issue of health as a human right is the right to dignity and care in the event that a person is already infected. A crucial method to prevent further spread of the disease once infection has set in is through early and voluntary testing. However, people will come forward for testing only if they know that it will be reliable and confidential and will not stigmatise them and alienate them from their social moorings, as happens regularly in the country at the present time. Testing also needs to be backed by respectful counselling about what lies ahead for the person if the test turns out positive, how to deal with others in the family and at the workplace, how to take care of his/her own health, and how to avoid infecting others. If people are not assured of this support, they would prefer to remain in ignorance about their HIV status. In many cases, however, people do not even have the choice of remaining ignorant. Most hospitals in the country make an HIV test mandatory for patients seeking admission for any surgery or childbirth. As the epidemic matures, sickness due to HIV infection is increasing, and positive persons visiting hospitals and doctors for health care are facing branding and humiliation, prohibitively high fees, or outright rejection.

The total lack of attention in medical colleges to training in ethics, their failure to sensitise their students to sexuality issues, remove irrational fears regarding HIV transmission, and promote HIV/AIDS as a professional area of choice, makes for a continuing dearth of doctors who have technical skills, social understanding and compassion in equal measure. The medical profession is yet to uphold the right of positive patients to skilled and respectful care.

When NGOs speak of HIV/AIDS as a human rights issue, therefore, they are critical of society condemning positive persons as not deserving of social justice or even humane social treatment. A human rights approach upholds the right to freedom from terror of being under a death sentence, the right to a good quality of life, and equality with non-positive persons on the one hand and with sufferers from other chronic diseases on the other. In terms of services, this means the right to professional ethics-driven pre-test and post-test counselling, good quality diagnostic facilities and drug treatment facilities that, together, can help the infected individual change his/her behaviour, remain integrated with his/her social networks, stay in reasonably good health and lead a productive life.

This does not imply that HIV be privileged above other more common preventable and high mortality diseases. Rather, the current human rights approach to HIV/AIDS has the potential to revolutionise the whole discourse on health as a human right, and move State and society towards institutional mechanisms that implement health rights.

Early HIV epidemiological research had showed up sexually active men and women with a large number of sexual partners and engaging in unprotected penetrative sex as the most vulnerable to STIs and HIV. Where these factors were found to be concentrated within certain definable groups, the groups came to be labelled 'high risk'. In the West, the virus first appeared and remained concentrated among white homosexual men. These men – educated and economically secure but socially stigmatised – responded with vigour. They 'came out' and acquired visibility, came together and organised themselves, learnt about the disease and the means of protection and, over time, were able to bring down the rates of infection among their communities. This instrument of awareness building known as 'peer education' – interactive learning within a group of equals – has since been held up by governments and grassroots organisations, national and international intervention agencies as the most effective means to bring about behaviour change in the context of HIV/AIDS. Behaviour change here refers to: reduced number of partners, consistent condom use and prompt treatment of sexually transmitted infections (STIs). Such change can bring down the rate of infection within vulnerable (high risk) groups, and simultaneously prevent the spread of the virus from these groups into the wider society. SANGRAM and Naz use peer education most effectively in their work.

Whether as a means of strengthening their role as civil society advocates, or to compensate for their own small scale, or to draw financial resources and persons with commitment to their activities, NGOs seek out a wide range of partnerships in society. None of the NGOs in this book make a virtue of ploughing lonely furrows, which is possibly one of the keys to their ability to weather periodic vicissitudes. All of them cast their net wide to draw in all sections of the society that are willing to support their cause. And, although they have a long way to go in this regard, a very important factor impelling these partnership-building exercises must be the felt need to replicate or multiply their own successes, or spread the positive lessons they have learnt. What might keep their efforts and scale limited is that each of these NGOs is not just involved in practical interventions, but also has a conceptual or ideological map of the road they have chosen to travel. This makes them feel committed to support or help initiate only those replication exercises that retain their core values, be it in terms of human rights, or continuum of prevention and care, rather than merely spawn clones for practical interventions minus the worldview.

Networking would seem to offer a middle path. Different NGOs can come together more easily on common platforms for specific actions, on a basis of equality, even though they may differ in the form they give to their shared zeal to change society, i.e., change the way people at large think and act. Advocacy thus becomes a common concern for all these NGOs. Most of the NGOs in the book are part of multiple networks at the regional, national and international levels, even as they are engaged in extending the reach of their programmes on the ground. What we have here are coalitions between middle class professionals and disadvantaged groups, between local NGOs and national networks, between individuals/community-based organisations/national networks and global networks.

Another instance of how the NGOs in this book 'network' is in their approach of working with existing actors and institutional structures in complementary (rather than confrontational) ways, thus synergising the maximum use of their own resources with those resources available outside. YRG CARE employs a wide-ranging referral network across south India that includes individual specialists, mainstream hospitals, and hospitals in the NGO/charitable structure, when treating their patients who come to them from all over the region. This helps them overcome the limitations of both distance and their own scale. SANGRAM's experience shows how community level work requires looking for common points of mutual interest among competing actors; the organisation works with both pimps and sex workers in its interventions. PREPARE's openness to working with managements, trade unions and workers enabled it to learn on its feet and strategise for maximum results, the most important being that of easing its own entry and acceptability in the factory. Despite its initial preference for approaching workers through the trade unions, it recognised that a strident trade union approach of fighting for workers' rights in the early stages of an intervention might neither benefit the workers in the long run, nor enlighten the managements. It was necessary to first educate all stakeholders about HIV/AIDS and its human rights dimensions, including the importance of managements refraining from carrying out HIV tests on workers as a condition for hiring or promoting them, and of workers learning the importance of changing their own sexual behaviours.

PREPARE's intervention also highlights the ambiguous outcomes that might result from interventions by outside NGOs, which calls for the capacity for flexibility and mid-course corrections on the part of NGOs. At the workplace, raising awareness about HIV/AIDS among managements may also result in the increased incidence of testing and refusal of employment opportunities. At such a point, NGOs may have to give way to trade unions to ensure that workers' rights are.not violated.

Would such 'organic' institutions – organisations of vulnerable people – then need continued support from outsider/middle class-led NGOs? At what point can NGOs begin to see themselves as no longer relevant as direct supports to the cause of the disadvantaged groups that they are empowering? The felt need of VAMP to continue to shelter under the umbrella of SANGRAM, or of the MSM support groups to remain under the protection of Naz, highlight the complexity in the evolution of vulnerable groups' capability to stand on their own. On this journey, they still continue to look to their middle class allies for support in negotiating a space for themselves in mainstream society, as well as in countering occasional assaults on their emerging identity as self-determined collectivities.

An important feature of NGOs is that they offer unique environments for the development of individual initiative, fulfilling careers and personal growth. In these small, intimate environments, there is scope for learning and decision-making that is not available in large formal organisations, to the usually young recruits who join NGOs. Paradoxically, these recruits acquire qualities – leadership, versatility – which then make them attractive to formal organisations.

For members of vulnerable communities themselves, NGO-like environments offer empowerment opportunities. For SANGRAM/VAMP, for example, condom distribution was a core activity, and their partnership with the government in the national programme was a source of legitimacy for them. But it was not enough, for if that were so, the VAMP activists would have been absorbed into the government programme that tried to poach them from SANGRAM. What was missing from the government programme, as they quickly learnt, was a role for them as equals; if anything, they were treated as the lowest level cogs in the huge government wheel. This brought them back to the SANGRAM/VAMP fold with doubled enthusiasm for NGO activism.

It is the smallness of scale of NGOs, of which scope for individual initiative is a component, that also makes face-to-face contact and support to vulnerable persons at an individual level a key element in their work. This is crucial in the context of HIV/AIDS. The sustained personal interaction that is part of the NGO work style helps them build 'communities' for consensual behaviour change and mutual support, out of otherwise atomised vulnerable people such as prostitutes or men who have sex with men or migrant workers. But this is not an easy task. In the absence of knowledge, discrimination can take place even within vulnerable communities. And education and counselling of all links in the chain are crucial, for example, SANGRAM's sex workers whose initial reaction to the positive women in their midst was one of rejection; those men engaging in same sex activity who see themselves as 'men' because they are penetrators, thus reflecting their own gender biases even within same sex interactions.

It is also crucial to remember that knowledge about HIV/AIDS does not make stigma go away. Nor indeed does the fact that 'information' is all around mean that people are 'seeing' it, or that they are interpreting the messages correctly. The notion that simply spreading information is enough to make for right action is a common middle class illusion, as evidenced by the employers and college principals that PREPARE and SANGRAM encountered, respectively, and the public interest advertisements that TARSHI analysed. Preparation of 'knowledge' and 'information' for the public requires prior understanding of the ways in which people think, see and receive. And changing the way people think and see, particularly helping them free themselves from behaviours that hurt themselves and others, requires learning through practice, and action within non-judgemental situations. Personal interaction with trained and skilled counsellors and with peers is very important in this exercise of being gently led to recognise one's own misconceptions and prejudices and how to discard them and change one's behaviour. In turn, stigmatised persons require the help of counsellors and peers to re-learn how to value themselves. The stigma attaching to HIV/AIDS has thrown up as never before the vital importance of counselling as an area of training and career choice, something that is very deficient in India. A major concern for NGOs must therefore be how to self-consciously keep strengthening the positive internal dynamics that makes them effective in the HIV/AIDS context: as environments within which initiative, autonomy, mutual responsibility and dignity can be learnt and practised and communicated to others.

Finally, all the NGOs in the book aim for independence, i.e., retaining their identity even if it requires them to stay small, and financial sustainability, i.e., raising their own money rather than depend solely on the vagaries and changing priorities of donor agencies. This is a particularly challenging task for NGOs doing treatment and care interventions that are capital and skill intensive, such as YRG CARE and Naz. NGO interventions, thus, have an in-built instability to them.

Part of the problem of instability arises from the fact that NGOs need to and do respond to stimuli, and keep expanding their roles as a result. Very often, as our case studies show, this happens because they find that nobody else is responding to an immediate issue. For example, when a positive woman was burnt to death in a village in PREPARE's project area, the incident received wide and sensational media coverage, but soon the matter disappeared from the media pages and was forgotten. It was an NGO – PREPARE – that quickly mustered the resources to throw itself into HIV/AIDS awareness raising among the communities in the area, in an effort to firefight the huge billowing smokescreen of stigma that had taken over. This led PREPARE into a whole new area of intervention with its spiralling spin-offs. The manner in which Naz, YRG CARE and the Lawyers Collective grew was similar in that one need that was identified led to a response, which in turn opened the doors to another set of needs, and so on. To some extent, such an expansion would appear to be an occupational hazard for NGOs, particularly when their internal environments are characterised by flexibility, open discussion as a basis for decision-making, regular progress reviews and willingness to change tracks in the interests of greater effectiveness. Expanding the activity profile could also be an instrument to back advocacy with service provision, for example, when Naz spread awareness about HIV/AIDS prevention among MSM, it generated a demand for testing. Naz found itself having to respond with setting up its own testing facility followed by a clinic for counselling and regular treatment because mainstream medical facilities denied MSM a confidential, non-stigmatising environment for care. For the Lawyers Collective to successfully steer the legal struggles of positive people, they had to conduct advocacy workshops for judges and lawyers and generally work to raise awareness about HIV/AIDS among related professional groups. Most often, as is evident from the case studies in this book, such impulses for expansion also emanate from the strong leadership figures that characterise all these NGOs, whose vision and considerable experience drive the organisation.

NGOs and/or their leaders do stop, from time to time, to introspect: Should they keep expanding? Would it be an efficient use of resources? Would it affect the quality of their services? Would they be able to sustain themselves financially? How to sustain enthusiasm among staff? How to cope with the impersonalisation and dilution of face-to-face mutual motivation that are bound to creep in with expansion? Leadership fatigue is also very real, but it is not an aspect that NGOs easily talk about. The creation of a second level leadership and the institutionalisation of these ventures is a theme that needs to be explored through a closer study.

To conclude, the NGOs involved in tackling the HIV/AIDS epidemic in India are different in some respects from NGOs in general. They tread a particularly difficult path, of which combating negativism is the most stressful component. The highly stigmatised environment and widespread misconceptions surrounding HIV/AIDS do not allow the easy sprouting of institutional innovations from the grassroots. It is a situation where exogenous interventions tend to play a more effective role. The innovators/founders of these interventions have been persons who are well trained, are grounded in the social/medical/legal terms of discourse on the subject, can hold their own in diverse forums, and to some extent have in them the makings of crusaders. It is an iterative process of weaving together the infrastructural and superstructural aspects of the HIV/AIDS epidemic. The founder-profile from the selection of NGOs in this book includes well-qualified medical practitioners, clinical and social psychologists, social workers and lawyers. All come from secure middle class backgrounds but are comfortable interacting on a daily basis with HIV positive persons and AIDS patients, they network with others in the NGO sector and in their own professional communities, and participate in debates and discussions around government policies and legislations. The case study narratives also reveal that they have the crusaders' grit in facing up to the challenges. Contrary to the general impression that there is a liberal flow of funds to support HIV/AIDS-related work, the case studies here point to a resource crunch. The financial sustainability of these institutions is far from guaranteed.

We had begun this introductory essay by describing cutting edge NGOs as institutional innovators who try and demonstrate the art of the possible. Four instruments emerge as practical models for replication and scaling up based on the experiences of the NGOs in this book.

One instrument is HIV/AIDS awareness raising in general and sexuality education in particular. NGOs use a variety of techniques that take counselling and face-to-face teaching and learning as their point of departure. Both in terms of the techniques themselves (including preparation of materials) and in terms of their application across virtually the entire spectrum of community-level and institutional locations, NGOs could act as catalysts to re-orient the mainstream.

A second and related instrument is peer education – so central to behavioural change within the context of the epidemic – with its principles of equality and interactive learning among those who share a common set of attributes, problems and challenges. Crafting consensual communities out of disparate individuals and bringing them together for mutual learning and support is something that these NGOs seem to have learnt to do. Spreading these skills across the society could prove effective in combating HIV/AIDS.

A third instrument relates to giving practical expression to the human right to dignity and citizenship for all, through legal reform and advocacy. Gross social inequalities and disadvantages offer breeding grounds for ever-newer forms of discrimination and inequities, as demonstrated by the manner in which HIV/AIDS hits harder at those who are socially disadvantaged.

The final instrument is the reinforcement of the right to safe and affordable health care for all as a right of critical social and political importance. The HIV/AIDS epidemic has sharpened the perspective on this right – respectful medical environments, mandatory universal precautions, affordable medicines – in an unprecedented manner.

SECTION ONE

Treatment and Care for People with HIV/AIDS

An Overview

Notwithstanding the controversy over the actual numbers of positive people in the country and their proportion vis-à-vis the general population, it is now fairly widely accepted that the number probably runs into several millions, and that India is among the three countries with the largest number of positive people in their populations.

Whereas in the early stages of the epidemic people with HIV had remained relatively invisible due to a combination of official and societal denial and general lack of sufficient public awareness about HIV, two decades into the epidemic those infected are becoming visible as patients in hospitals across the country – whether as pregnant women, or as victims of TB, or as patients requiring treatment and/or surgery for myriad problems just as do non-HIV persons – due to the practice of mandatory testing adopted by most hospitals. The price of this visibility is the stigma, discrimination and, often, outright rejection that these patients face when they seek care for even routine ailments or maternity-related care. HIV/AIDS has thus forced its way into public consciousness as a prominent and expanding part of the social fabric. Even as approaches to HIV prevention continue to remain gravely flawed nearly three decades into the epidemic, the issue of treatment and care of people already infected with the virus is emerging as a major issue in the country and as something that will have to be planned for by the State in collaboration with the private and NGO sectors.

The rapid depletion of immunity that is the hallmark of the HIV virus is a feature that makes it unique as a disease where the immune system, which is supposed to defend the body against pathogens, is itself attacked. This renders people living with HIV/AIDS (PLWHAs) more susceptible than victims of other communicable diseases to a variety of 'opportunistic infections'. These infections may be recurrent and/or concurrent, and could range from simple to complex. The most commonly occurring opportunistic infections in India are tuberculosis, candidiasis, bacterial pneumonia, herpes zoster, skin diseases, etc.

Although HIV itself is incurable, most of the above-listed specific infections are treatable. It is a scientifically proven fact that timely and appropriate treatment of opportunistic infections could improve the quality of life of positive persons and retain their usefulness to family and community. It prevents depletion of immunity, keeps down the viral load, and delays the escalation of HIV into AIDS and therefore premature death. From the public health point of view, reduction in the viral load helps check the further spread in the society of infections like TB that are already rampant in the society. Treatment with drugs for opportunistic infections works best when it is accompanied by good nutrition (an essential accompaniment for all treatments, whether one is HIV positive or not) and psychological support (that helps patients stay optimistic, and comply with the requirements of the therapy they are undergoing, again common to all long-duration therapies). There are also the debilitating effects of other common infections – water, food and airborne infections and, particularly, diarrhoeal diseases – that are a routine part of life in India, particularly if one is in a situation of economic and social disadvantage. These too could affect HIV positive persons particularly badly if they do not receive prompt or proper treatment.

The other aspect of treatment of positive persons is the timely identification of the person's readiness for starting on anti-retroviral drugs. The advent of combination ART (anti-retroviral therapy) in 1996 has made a qualitative difference to the issue of treatment and care. Combination ART is a cocktail of three anti-retroviral (ARV) drugs mixed together to prevent drug resistance. It brings down the viral load and boosts the immune system and delays further damage to it. It thus holds out the real possibility of improving the quality of life and longevity of those already infected. One form of ART is available as Post-Exposure Prophylaxis (PEP). If taken within three hours of exposure or at the most within 72 hours of a needle stick injury (accidental prick from an infected injection needle or surgery equipment to health personnel or home-based carers of positive patients) or accidental sexual relations, or criminal risk exposure (such as rape), it can protect the person from infection. Since research into various ART drug formulations is an ongoing exercise, specifications may undergo change from time to time. The important thing is that for the first time due to ART, HIV/AIDS is no longer the immutable death sentence that it once was. It is possible for people to live fairly long lives just as they would in the case of any chronic disease, provided that ART is administered in a timely manner. Apart from its humanitarian impact, the strongest argument in support of ART is that the knowledge that HIV/AIDS is a treatable disease may act as a spur to voluntary testing and treatment and, through the effect of breaking the cycle of transmission, have a significant impact upon public health.

ARVs, however, have several drawbacks. They are very expensive and, as they have to be taken life-long, they are beyond the reach of most persons. Secondly, they are highly toxic and could cause pain and unfamiliar forms of discomfort. Further, ARV drugs require strict adherence to complex protocols for administration – the number and combination of doses, the time of day for intake, etc. – without which drug resistance could set in. They also require regular monitoring tests in order to fine tune further administration and, importantly, check for drug resistance. For all of the above, patients need to be supported by medical practitioners well versed in ARV treatment, sustained by counselling, and family (or peer) support through the difficult treatment process, so that they do not default on intake and develop drug resistance. The therapy also presupposes great attention to nutrition and general well-being which, too, is costly. All these features pose major obstacles to ARV treatment in the Indian context, particularly among low-income communities. Added problems come from the burden of stigma and the attendant secrecy and, very frequently, loss of even family support and attendant social isolation, conditions that are not very conducive for patient morale, especially where complex and long duration treatment regimens are concerned. Finally, ART is not a substitute for continued condom use. If patients on ART become complacent and lapse back into risky, i.e., unprotected sexual behaviour, it could result in the continuing spread of the virus, this time of drug-resistant varieties. Recent and ongoing research points to the crucial need for patients on ARV drugs to combine it with condom use or effective preventive behaviour for the true public health gains of ARV therapies to be realised.

The treatment and care of positive persons using anti-retroviral drugs is, therefore, a complex challenge calling for a high degree of medical and counselling skills and collaboration and trust between patients and providers.

Poor patients desperately seeking treatment tend to make frequent crossovers between self-medication, the government health services, and a wide range of unregulated fee-charging modern and traditional private providers, including quacks who proclaim miracle cures for problems like HIV. Patients choose their kind of provider based on their changing assessment of their own health condition and the affordability and perceived efficacy of providers in the open market. Often, these decisions are attended by indebtedness, as family members forego wages and/or sell assets in the search for cures. Despite these efforts, HIV positive persons who approach the formal health system with a problem are at a greater disadvantage than sufferers of other communicable diseases. Medical professionals – doctors, nurses, ward boys, *ayahs* (women helpers) – have an excessive fear of becoming infected themselves, a huge factor leading to the denial of even routine care to people identified as positive. For the same reason, they are afraid that the presence of positive patients – as outpatients or in-patients – could bring disrepute to their medical establishment. Paradoxically, therefore, HIV positive persons who may be more in need of periodic medical treatment and care than sufferers of most other communicable diseases are the ones who are most denied this when they go forth to seek care.

It is a scientific fact that the observance of universal precautions can effectively safeguard health sector actors from accidental infection in the medical environment, and that prompt resort to PEP (Post-Exposure Prophylaxis) in the event of an accident can provide near total protection. The unwillingness of medical professionals to heed these scientific findings is moored in a more fundamental sociological factor. This is the enormous and irrational stigma and discrimination that is directed against people who are identified as positive. The roots of this stigma lie principally in the widespread association of HIV with some kind of sexual 'misconduct', and an immediate negative judgement regarding the 'character' of the person concerned. For instance, treatment-seeking married women are invariably asked derisively by health personnel whether they are sex workers. And, when socially aware positive persons take the initiative to inform the attending medical professional of their positive status in order that the latter may observe due precautions, they become objects of public curiosity and rejection.

Aggressive public policies are required that mandate primary orientation and periodic retraining of all medical professionals in the scientific and behavioural aspects of HIV/AIDS. Equally, government policy must make universal precautions and prompt access to PEP mandatory in all government and private hospitals. If these measures are properly enforced, fear and stigmatisation of care seekers may be expected to diminish. When hospital authorities are compelled to make available money and training for the purchase and correct use of these life-saving measures, the medical environment will become less risky for both health staff and patients.

The best instances hitherto of treatment and care of positive patients that combine the qualities of patient and family counselling, compassion and non-discriminatory behaviour by health personnel, thorough medical knowledge and training, observance of universal precautions, and affordable treatment have been in the NGO sector. Here, dedication and idealism have been able to overcome the impediments that private and public facilities are more prone to fall prey to. Most often, these NGOs focus on effective treatment for opportunistic infections, and administer ARV drugs simply as a strategic and time-bound humanitarian panacea. ARVs are not given in the manner of a life-long treatment, but just so that despairing families may hold together for a little while longer. The 'best practice' in medical treatment and care under Indian conditions may be summed up thus: respectful and confidential counselling to help patients and their families understand the new and unfamiliar disease; competent medical treatment that can give patients temporary reprieve from suffering and extend their productive lives at least until they feel they have discharged their family and social obligations; a special focus on women patients in general, and medical assistance in the case of a pregnancy or delivery; and, lowering the levels of stigma and fear within the medical environment.

The following chapter presents the case of one such best practice. Today, YRG CARE is upheld both nationally and internationally as a model centre for comprehensive HIV/AIDS care, and as a case of 'best practice' that offers lessons for other aspiring treatment and care centres in similar resource-poor settings in the voluntary sector.

The Continuum of Treatment and Care
The YRG CARE Model

SUNITI SOLOMON

YRG CARE in Chennai was one of the earliest groups in the country to plunge into HIV/AIDS work. Working steadily and learning on its feet, it today brings together an unusually broad array of skills, services and networks that together offer HIV patients, particularly in the state of Tamil Nadu and in southern India in general, the opportunity to cope with the disease and achieve some measure of control over their lives. Since its inception, YRG CARE's mission has been to provide an affordable, client-centred continuum of care that not only serves the changing needs of HIV positive clients through all stages of the disease and treatment, but also addresses the prevention and support needs of their families and others affected by HIV/AIDS in their midst. In addition, the organisation fulfills a larger role within the community of building prevention awareness, promoting safe and responsible sexual behaviour, reducing stigmatising attitudes towards people living with HIV/AIDS, and advocating policies that protect the rights of those affected by the epidemic.

The hallmark of YRG CARE is to be found in three features that it has evolved self-consciously. One is its self-identity as a learning organisation, constantly combining scientific research with grassroots-level interactive educational approaches. A second is its client-centred approach, whereby it has consistently been governed by its clients' vulnerabilities, experiences and needs. This has meant being open to growth in new and unplanned directions. The perception of each new client-need or vulnerability has led to the addition of new services, and these in turn have often snowballed to reveal yet other needs. YRG CARE's third feature is its extensive referral network with other medical institutional facilities and individual providers for managing clinical and psychosocial support, and with other NGOs and People Living with HIV/AIDS (PLWHAs) networks for emotional and social support.

Early beginnings

The story of YRG CARE began in 1986, simultaneously with the onset of the HIV epidemic in India. I was then working as a microbiologist at the Madras Medical College in Chennai (formerly Madras), and it was in the course of my work there that, for the first time in India, we were able to document and confirm the presence of HIV in blood samples drawn from Tamil Nadu-based sex workers. Like many others in the country at the time, I too had believed that HIV was a disease of the West and of homosexuals that would never come to India. However, this first confirmation of the presence of the virus in the country exploded that myth, and my world was never to be the same again. Subsequent events seemed to take on a life of their own, as I found myself borne aloft on a huge learning wave. As I worked to educate myself about the scientific and social dimensions of the disease, the enormity of HIV's potential for spread and devastation in a country of India's dimensions began to dawn on me.

I observed that two major scenarios had begun unfolding in my immediate environment. One was widespread ignorance, complacency, indifference and misconceptions, the common perception being that HIV was a disease that affected only those at the 'margins' of Indian society, such as visiting foreigners, sex workers, and 'immoral' people in general. The other was that not many medical professionals were willing to accept the existence of the disease and its sexual mode of transmission. The associated moral overtones meant absence of willingness among these professionals to learn about the disease and to put together meaningful responses to it, responses that ought to be based on scientific understanding and professional skills. In my own state of Tamil Nadu as well as elsewhere in the country, official and popular responses to the new disease veered from casual dismissal of the disease, to calls for the imprisonment of sex workers, to confused and contradictory public 'messages' about the nature of the disease and means for its prevention.

As my understanding about the disease grew, I felt compelled to intervene. Initially, this intervention was within my own area of specialisation, microbiology. But HIV was too multifaceted a disease to permit of such a restricted involvement. As the stream of people (mostly young) now coming to my laboratory with questions, doubts, fears and requests for HIV testing continued to swell, I found myself swept into the role of advocate for HIV prevention. Every day new and unfamiliar roles awaited me that took me far beyond that of scientist and medical professional. Once having decided to respond to the bewildering multiplicity of demands, I found myself having to acquire skills that I would have never imagined I would exercise as a medical professional: counsellor to individuals and their families; educator and interventionist with schools, colleges and employers; networker with other scientific institutions and lay groups both within and outside the country; organiser, popular writer, fund raiser; and advisor to governmental, international and funding organisations.

Testing

Following the initial realisation that the virus had become naturalised in India and in Chennai in particular, the first task that our laboratory at the Madras Medical College took on was to track the levels of infection in Tamil Nadu and its trends among the earliest identified 'high risk' groups, including commercial sex workers and patients presenting themselves at sexually transmitted diseases (STD) clinics in the public sector.

A major hurdle we faced was the non-availability of testing kits with which to check the HIV status of these patients. We were fortunate to be able to enter into a collaborative arrangement with the other handful of pioneering scientists working on HIV at the Christian Medical College in nearby Vellore. Initially, we carried out our tests in Vellore, but soon we were training our own laboratory personnel, using testing kits borrowed from Vellore. We were now the new AIDS Research Cell within the Madras Medical College, and one of the earliest research groups of its kind in Tamil Nadu. When the Indian Council of Medical Research (ICMR) set up its Sentinel Surveillance Programme in 1986, we were an obvious candidate for inclusion as one of its affiliated centres. The funding from the ICMR went some way towards solving the immediate problem of availability of kits. But the AIDS Research Cell's activities went far beyond the confines of the ICMR programme. As our efforts to spread awareness about HIV in Tamil Nadu society at large grew over the next few years, so too did the demand for testing. We tried not to allow infrastructural obstacles to come in the way of our work by establishing early links with local pharmaceutical firms that had by now begun to manufacture testing kits, and persuading them to donate free kits to the Cell.

It was not long before the realisation dawned on us that while the availability of testing was helping raise all-round awareness about the disease, it was not sufficient. For the individuals who voluntarily came forward to be tested, the laboratory technology was the proverbial tip of the iceberg beneath which seethed social, cultural and human ramifications that were as contentious and fluid as the medical dimensions themselves. The trauma of those who tested positive, and the possible impact of this knowledge on their life plans and social relationships, all called for one-on-one counselling. My colleagues and I in the AIDS Research Cell (which was still part of the Microbiology Department of the Madras Medical College at the time) were compelled to arm ourselves with counselling skills. We thus became the first HIV counselling service in Tamil Nadu. The transformative role that this foray into counselling played in my own growth was nothing short of revolutionary. My involvement with the virus and the people in its net was threatening to become a life-long affair. HIV counselling was pushing me into plumbing the depths of a communication process that I had never imagined existed. I began to realise that the manner in which this process was steered could make the difference between life and death for the sufferers. As far as I was aware, no other disease before this paralleled HIV in this regard.

Pre-test counselling at the AIDS Research Cell consisted (and continues to consist) of helping individuals understand: basic facts about the disease; the need for testing based on ascertaining risk-related behaviour; the test itself – the waiting period for results, window period, re-testing if negative, possible fallouts should the test prove positive –; how social support networks could be harnessed; possible preventive strategies; and how to move towards behavioural change. In the event of the individual testing positive, post-test counselling calls for even greater sensitivity and emotional support. There needs to be detailed discussion between counsellor and patient covering: support of family and friends; understanding the difference between HIV and AIDS, and how to actively participate in self-care so as to prolong the productive years; dealing with sexual partners including revealing HIV status; understanding and coming to terms with the arguments for and against marriage and starting a family; safe sex methods and the crucial importance of preventing further spread; diet and nutrition; opportunistic infections; and treatment and caring for oneself in sickness.

Today, our counselling services go beyond the individual to include marital and couple counselling, antenatal and nutritional counselling, family counselling, counselling of other persons in the support system, and grief counselling.

Public education

The AIDS Research Cell's steady surveillance activities in Tamil Nadu were revealing galloping trends in HIV infection rates. Five per cent of the first 100 HIV cases coming to the Cell, alone, were students. On the basis of both our surveillance activities and from among those coming in for voluntary testing, we found that young people (16-24 years) consistently formed a distinctive subset of those testing positive. A huge ignorance about sexuality in general and the virus in particular was evident from the questions, doubts and uncertainties expressed by the individuals coming to the AIDS Research Cell. All these brought home to us the realisation that a laboratory-based approach, i.e., waiting for people to come to us, would not halt the spread of the infection in any way.

In 1991, the AIDS Research Cell metamorphosed into the AIDS Resource Group. Still under the umbrella of the Madras Medical College, it now became a multi-disciplinary group consisting of a microbiologist (myself), serologist, blood bank officer, clinician, STD specialist and psychiatrist. Our objective was to undertake a grassroots engagement with the emerging epidemic. Our first port of call was young people. Fanning out to schools and colleges, the group engaged in broad-based awareness raising programmes through debates, discussions, plays and talks and, gradually, into question-and-answer based sex education sessions for separate groups of boy and girl students. To help lift the taboos on discussion of sex and sexuality issues, we held initial workshops with principals of educational institutions and their Parent-Teacher Associations. Although initially resistant, these opinion makers were won over.

Our group was equally proactive in its engagement with the general public. We initiated panel discussions and question and answer sessions on radio and television, organised events around World AIDS Day, and designed programmes specially tailored to the needs of and requests from other NGOs, clubs, societies, associations like the Rotary Club, and commercial and industrial undertakings.

Group members also went out among a range of special interest groups: religious groups (including church groups), taxi, auto and truck drivers, industrial workers' groups, associations and unions, commercial sex workers, STD patients, prison and remand home inmates, and slum colonies. We conducted workshops for English and Tamil print journalists, for senior administrators and policy makers of the state and municipal governments.

The focus in all the programmes was: raising awareness about the disease, advocating the rights of positive people to compassionate and caring treatment by society, and the need for public and private agencies to work together towards planning and implementing policies for the control of the epidemic. Within a month of the group's existence, we launched a monthly newsletter specifically targeted to NGOs, emerging AIDS service organisations (like the AIDS Research Foundation of India in Chennai), and other individuals and groups involved in AIDS-related activities in India and abroad. Through all of the above, we continued to focus special attention on the youth – both in school and college, and outside of institutional structures – as the most vulnerable section, on the threshold of adulthood, open to sexual experimentation, and lacking in access to accurate and friendly information about sex. The language of communication was at all times both English and Tamil. And the group built on the advantage that all of its members were doctors and, therefore, were seen as authoritative and acceptable by all sections and strata of Tamil Nadu society.

As the public educational process advanced, we carried out systematic reviews of our programmes (through KAP studies) to improve upon presentation content and communication techniques. We engaged newer batches of students and ever-widening circles of youth in our communication programmes. Other groups, too, came to be included, based on the felt needs of clients coming in for testing. For example, as more and more employed young persons tested positive and required rehabilitation in their workplaces, senior level welfare officers and industry personnel managers, factory owners and their staff, and associations of commerce and industry became an important target group for education and negotiation. The objective was to remove discriminatory attitudes at the workplace and help organisations frame policies that accommodated care and support systems for infected employees. Thus, from the initial testing and surveillance in 1986, to the expansion into counselling, to the launching of public education programmes from the start of the 1990s, the work of the group had expanded exponentially.

As awareness spread and people volunteered to be tested, their medical needs began to press for attention as yet another area for intervention. We had already identified medical professional groups such as the Indian Medical Association, blood banking staff, technicians and nurses, general practitioners, personnel from medical colleges and private and public hospitals, both within the city of Chennai and throughout the state, as an important audience for awareness-raising talks and workshops since they were among the least informed about the disease, its prevention and treatment, and among the most unwilling to engage with patients who happened to be HIV positive. It was little use telling people that they had tested positive, counselling and educating them, and then leaving them at the mercy of a medical environment that rejected them when they needed medical help. To wait for an uncertain future when the medical community would become responsive, did not seem realistic.

The AIDS Resource Group was, admittedly, outgrowing its disciplinary and organisational configuration. A different action format was called for, a dedicated centre that combined medical testing and treatment, and social services. This involved breaking new ground with no precedent within the country, either in the NGO or public sectors. And there was no time to be lost. I did what was most immediately available to me; I gathered together support from within my own family, and in 1993 the Y.R.Gaitonde Centre for AIDS Research and Education (YRG CARE) was formally born as an NGO, a public charity, and a unit of the Y.R.Gaitonde Medical, Educational and Research Foundation (a family Foundation). The new research foundation provided the needed autonomy and singular focus for engaging full-time in AIDS-related work in all its aspects. Its mission was to work towards a world where people with HIV/AIDS and their families would live in dignity, and where further spread of infection would be halted. It saw its niche as responding to the needs of people who were not receiving care and support or education and information about HIV within the south India region.

Setting in motion the continuum of care

By 1993, HIV positive persons were already showing up in hospitals and clinics with stubborn opportunistic infections. The poor, particularly, tended to arrive at a medical facility only when the disease was already in its final stages.

As sick HIV patients began to stream into YRG CARE, we realised that we had to intensify our awareness programmes for medical and paramedical and hospital personnel in Chennai city and in the southern states generally. Almost all the patients coming to YRG CARE – and particularly those from outside Chennai – had earlier done the rounds of mainstream health care facilities. And they had faced discrimination and rejection the moment their HIV status became known. Tackling the issue of discrimination against HIV infected people within formal health care settings, therefore, assumed significant priority in our list of objectives. Equally, we recognised that even sympathetic health care providers were unable to treat positive patients due to their lack of accurate scientific knowledge about the disease and treatment possibilities. Many of the patients coming to YRG CARE for treatment had also been to quacks who either wrongly diagnosed them or offered them spurious cures. Either way, patients found that seeking care resulted in depletion of their scarce monetary reserves. It also heightened their sense of hopelessness.

An important aspect of patients' health-seeking behaviour was that irrespective of whether patients went from one provider to another, or travelled from other parts of south India to YRG CARE, a significant proportion of their costs (including costs of accompanying care-givers) went into transport. This clearly pointed to the need for more decentralised care facilities within the state. Networking and partnerships between medical institutions and professionals appeared to be the only way forward in coping with the huge numbers of HIV positive people requiring care.

With all this in view, we launched a periodic publication – *Wrap Up* – that summarised new developments in HIV/AIDS care and support that were relevant to the Indian context. This publication was distributed to over 3000 physicians and care providers working in NGO, government and private institutions throughout south India. We no longer print this publication with the increase in government training programmes and easy access to information over the Net. YRG CARE also offers professional training in HIV and related fields to doctors and paramedics who seek such training. Medical interns from local medical colleges are taken in to give them first hand experience of working with people living with HIV/AIDS (PLWHAs).

Over time, this strategy has borne fruit. We have built mutually supportive networks with other institutions and providers within the state. Within Chennai itself, since 1995, we have an impressive consortium of consultants in premier specialty institutions to whom we refer our patients whenever necessary. In this manner, we continue to work towards mainstreaming HIV/AIDS, even while our own sphere of operations remains within the NGO sector.

Our decision to incorporate treatment and care early in our HIV/AIDS-related work arose out of our observation that HIV positive people faced two very real and basic obstacles. One obstacle was the frequent opportunistic infections that they were prone to. Opportunistic infections in HIV positive patients have to be treated differently than among non-HIV patients. However, since most of the providers lacked the skills to make correct diagnosis for HIV-related opportunistic infections and offer effective treatment, families tended to lose both valuable time and scarce financial resources due to their fruitless chase from one provider to another. This was true irrespective of whether or not the providers were 'formal' doctors. The delay in treatment escalated the progression of the virus. Since at the time no drugs existed to treat the virus itself, the result was speedy deterioration and finally the death of the patient. Besides having to cope with illness and death of a family member, the experience of care-seeking pushed several families deeply into debt. The other obstacle that positive patients faced in care-seeking was the appallingly stigmatising treatment meted out to HIV patients in all mainstream medical facilities, public and private.

For YRG CARE, the overarching concern was the right of people to know about HIV/AIDS, about their own status in relation to it, and how to cope with their condition when their health began to give way. Equally, it was their right to be treated with dignity and respect in the medical environment whenever they approached it for the solution of a health problem and to be able to lead a better quality of life. To this end, we identified our challenge as one of offering at YRG CARE a confidential and respectful environment for people to talk about their problems and concerns, and prompt and effective treatment for opportunistic infections and their complications. At this stage of development of knowledge about the disease, the key to fighting the epidemic, according to us, was to prevent the spread of HIV infection through education, testing, preventing opportunistic infections through prophylactic treatment, or timely cure of these infections, and counselling about nutrition and lifestyles.

However, meeting the steadily escalating demand for funds for doing treatment and care work posed huge problems. In the initial years of YRG CARE's existence – 1993 to 1997 – none of the established donors were willing to fund care and support for positive people, focused as they were on prevention. True, anti-retroviral drugs had still not come into the Indian market. But even the crucial (and more affordable) role of combining prompt attention to opportunistic infections with nutrition and family counselling – tools that were already in existence – was not recognised. Even procuring a physical space for the new organisation and setting up in-patient facilities proved to be a difficult task, given the generally discriminatory attitudes towards HIV.

In 1997, a small grant from AUSAID made it possible to recruit full-time medical personnel. It also enabled YRG CARE to begin clinical research in association with U.S. universities, notably Brown University. This opened the windows for negotiation with these collaborators for access to diagnostic kits, as well as drugs for common opportunistic infections. Research projects have also helped support staff salaries. In a sense, research collaborations have become a tool through which we have been able to keep our medical care services afloat. The institutional review board, an ethics committee comprising of leading clinicians, researchers and social and legal advocates within YRG CARE, ensures complete transparency in the matter of these research collaborations. We assure safety of patient participants in research studies at all times, and do not carry out any testing of experimental drugs, devices or procedures on patients.

Other developments that took place in 1997 added synergy to the above-described developmental spurt. We were able to secure premises for YRG CARE in the campus of the Voluntary Health Services, a charitable medical facility in Chennai. With this our physical stability and expansion of our facilities became somewhat assured. We renovated the existing dilapidated leprosy block and converted it into a 24-bed ward for actively ill patients with complications of opportunistic infections and needing intensive care. Other services on the premises consisted of a walk-in testing and counselling facility, a family support centre, and a women's clinic and paediatric clinic which together offer day care, hospital-based care and home care. With this, YRG CARE became among the first organisations in the country to offer scientific treatment and care for HIV/AIDS, to in-patients and outpatients, men, women and children.

The fact that treatment and care had become our core activity did not mean the end of our public education activities. We have strengthened and streamlined our prevention programmes for adolescents and youth using slide shows, small group discussions, participatory methods, and peer education. Our community-based awareness programmes have continued, particularly focusing on urban slums. The focused approach has been extended to include specially tailored awareness programmes for specific populations, as for example prison populations, through creating the conditions for voluntary anonymous screening. We have also acquired a reputation for training instructors in sex education, HIV/AIDS and counselling. YRG CARE is a lead organisation in the Tamil Nadu State AIDS Control Society (TANSACS)-UNICEF School AIDS Education Programme, which also integrates with the District Institute of Education and Training centres in Tamil Nadu to provide training programmes. Other public activities include a training and mentorship programme in clinical and psychosocial management of HIV. The YRG CARE Learning Resources Unit (LRU), with its wide collection of scientific and popular learning resources, is freely accessible to the public. Finally, there are the popular, priced books and pamphlets in English and Tamil that we publish periodically about HIV, its prevention, care and management within the Indian context. The needs and concerns of the wide cross-section of people that we interact with in the course of counselling and public education provide the impetus for these publications.

Research capacity

Above all, it is building scientific capacity that has been at the core of YRG CARE's own developmental agenda. Although engaged at the grassroots in the cultural and social dimensions of the disease, the group has fiercely sustained its identity as a scientific group and continues to maintain formal and informal communication links with the scientific community, both within the country and internationally. Evidence of this is our openness to forging collaborative research linkages with other medical groups both in India and overseas. One of our early programmes was medical and drug experimentation on herbal medicines for HIV in collaboration with some scientific departments in Chennai. Other themes for research collaboration over the years have been: the progression of the disease in high-risk populations, opportunistic infections in HIV patients, microbicides for women, and mother-to-child transmission. YRG CARE actively participates in ongoing scientific debates through research articles published in peer reviewed international and national medical journals (68 papers as of February 2005), and participation in national and international scientific meetings. Our considerable body of publications arising out of our clinical and social research, and our own statistics and experiences, also provide the basis for the organisation's investment of time and effort in participation in state, national, and international meetings and conferences. Through this engagement, we aspire to influence the adoption of more appropriate policies in relation to prevention, care and support for people living with HIV/AIDS (PLWHAs).

The focus on treatment and care

The comprehensive prevention and prevention-related training and public education services to the community, community-based organisations and the medical and scientific community described above constitute an inseparable part of YRG CARE's continuum of care. Another significant component is the provision of comprehensive quality treatment and care for those living with HIV. Two inalienable elements in this provision are: an environment that is compassionate, confidential and affordable, and a mechanism for regular follow-up.

Today, over 7,000 people living with HIV/AIDS along with their families throughout south India are being regularly counselled, treated and monitored by YRG CARE's comprehensive services. YRG CARE was the first organisation in the country – in the government and non-governmental sectors – to implement a client-centred integrated model of care which includes: early detection, confidential psychosocial counselling, diet and nutrition, medical interventions in the form of low cost symptom control, effective treatment of opportunistic infections, reducing mother-to-child transmission wherever possible through judicious provision of anti-retroviral drugs (ever since these became available) to pregnant mothers, providing ARV drugs to patients who can afford it, and the practice of universal precautions by YRG CARE staff and family carers. A team of six full-time doctors, thirteen nurses and three paramedics offer care. A dental clinic also provides services as part of the day care centre. We are one of the four sites under the Global Fund Programme involving public-private partnerships for enhancing anti-retroviral therapy based upon a graduated cost recovery mechanism which involves four tiers; tier one pays 100 per cent, tier two pays 75 per cent, tier three pays 50 per cent, while tier four gets free anti-retrovirals in addition to monitoring.

The doctors, nurses and paramedics also provide home-based care, which includes both medical care and psychosocial support. This service was begun in 1994 for those who were terminally ill, or pregnant, or who lived within a 30 kilometre radius of the hospital. It is also available to wealthy and influential patients who do not wish to publicly access the YRG CARE hospital. As part of the home-based care programme, a senior nurse makes regular visits to the family, and visits are made by a doctor whenever necessary. The home care team travel by auto rickshaw and are never in uniform, and patient confidentiality is respected at all times.

Today, patients come to our facilities from everywhere in the country, but more so from other parts of south India. Many of these patients have to travel long distances to reach us. Given this, we recognise the crucial importance of ensuring that patients always have somewhere to go to for treatment. One of our ongoing attempts, therefore, is to constantly build and maintain a viable referral network. Referral is also offered wherever there are gaps in service at YRG CARE itself, and whenever patients request it. An important concomitant of this process of referral is our attempts to advocate for higher standards of HIV patient care in other health facilities in the region, of which consistent adoption of universal precautions at all mainstream medical institutions in Tamil Nadu and the southern region is a central component. In the absence of precautions, health workers in these institutions have a genuine fear of contracting the virus, and hence tend to reject patients or stigmatise them. The absence of observance of universal precautions is one of the stumbling blocks that come in the way of HIV positive patients accessing mainstream medical facilities. YRG CARE's referral network also offers patients other support services such as legal assistance, employment assistance, insurance, etc., with the help of volunteer professionals.

A touchstone of our patient policy is to keep our services affordable. Our price structure, based on income, follows a three-tier pricing scheme. Outpatients tend to be charged at the highest tier. In-patients are generally charged at the middle tier, reflecting the fact that sicker patients have lower incomes (and fewer support services or facilities at home). Low-income clients are charged at the lowest tier. For the poorest, services are free, except for a token amount of Rs. 50 per day for in-patients.

Despite our efforts in this regard, seeking care could be crippling for an HIV patient. What increases the financial burden for the patient are the other costs associated with care-seeking. A recent study of patients accessing the facilities at YRG CARE found that transport costs for patients and carers (including food and lodging during the trip) could amount to almost 30 per cent of the direct costs of illness. Medical costs constitute the remaining 70 per cent. The study also found that the direct costs of HIV/AIDS illness – including both medical and non-medical expenses – among those coming to YRG CARE, amount to an average of almost 50 per cent of household income, going up to around 80 per cent for patients at a more advanced stage of the disease. The striking feature was that low-income households spent the highest proportion of their income (82 per cent) on the direct costs involved in combating HIV/AIDS. Another effect on household income/expenditure is due to the fact that people living with HIV/AIDS take time off from work, or find less physically demanding jobs, or reduce the number of hours that they work, or stop working altogether due to frequent episodes of illness. The dual effect of loss of income due to loss of work and costs of treatment is the high prevalence of indebtedness among PLWHA and their families. But even more than loss of work, it is treatment-seeking – amounting to as much as 67 per cent of the debt burden, and a sizeable proportion of this consumed by transport costs – that lays patients low. Despite the above grim picture, one valuable finding was that for many of the patients the treatment experience at YRG CARE helped them improve their capacity to work. Their absenteeism from work fell from 43 days on average (during the six months prior to seeking YRG CARE's services) to 14 days (at the end of the first year of care at YRG CARE).

Looking back, looking ahead

The fact that YRG CARE is currently able to meet only a fraction of the felt needs of people with HIV, as well as the findings of the study referred to above, prompted us to begin to explore the possibility of decentralising treatment, through setting up treatment centres at many more locations in the southern region. Decentralising the YRG CARE model of continuum of care would not simply be a matter of enlarging the YRG CARE programme or transplanting it in another place. We would need to be guided by the locations as well as the potential partners who would have their own specific organisational cultures, resources, needs, strengths and weaknesses. What we saw as important was to replicate the *concept*. This involved transferring the core values of patient-centred care: respect for patient dignity and confidentiality and involvement of communities and families.

With some seed money and technical support from the International HIV/AIDS Alliance – an international NGO –, we selected our scale-up partners from four sites, one each in the four southern states of Tamil Nadu, Andhra Pradesh, Kerala and Karnataka. As a first step, we worked to identify the partners' own needs and goals. We then developed a training and capacity building programme tailored to each site; the programme was conducted by my staff. The programme is currently underway, and it is too early to evaluate its efficacy.

For YRG CARE itself, a major and continuing challenge is how to maintain a regular inflow of funds to sustain the prevention-care continuum that has thrown open an ever-expanding canvas of activities and increased public demand for quality HIV/AIDS-related services. Another allied challenge is how to sustain the quality of our services.

One of the policy suggestions that emerged from the study cited earlier is that YRG CARE increase its paying patient load as a means of strengthening its financial viability. However, the option of taking in ever-increasing patient loads – already a natural pressure upon the organisation – poses for us the issue of quality sustainability. Reconciling high quality of care for all with affordable care for poor patients is a big challenge, in which the watchword is vigilance. Sustaining quality entails rigorous training and retraining of all clinical staff, including other forms of support such as partnering new entrants with more experienced staff. The organisation is conscious of the need to guard against any lapse on that front.

One of the ways in which we are trying to respond to the challenge of financial sustainability is to consciously and doggedly try to develop the skills to identify, nurture, and efficiently and imaginatively husband a diverse source of funds, each small but important. The mechanisms we have fallen back upon are collaborations, linkages and networking, and our partners in this have been the scientific community within India and overseas, other NGOs, international donors, and members of the public. Core programme grants form the bedrock of our financial base. Collaborative research grants, mostly through tie-ups with leading U.S. universities sharing common research interests, bring in much-needed funds, equipment, and scientific skill enhancement. The research and clinical internships that we offer to students seeking hands-on field experience contribute their mite in the form of student fees. Donations from pharmaceutical firms, fees from consulting assignments and training fees have been other sources since the early days of the organisation. Innovative community-based fund raising programmes complete the financial portfolio. For example, a simple source of funds for nutrition of patients, which also carries the message of YRG CARE's work to the general public, is our '365 Good Friends Programme'. Under this programme, members of the public are encouraged to make fixed annual donations in the name of loved ones, alive or deceased. On their respective birthdays or special days, special and nutritious food is cooked and served to all patients, both in-patient and outpatient. YRG CARE's goal is to secure firm commitments from the public for all 365 days of the year. In this manner, an important organisational cost is met. And, through the imaginative use of a culturally familiar symbol – feeding strangers in the name of a loved one –, members of the public are drawn in as donors to the organisation and as supporters of HIV/AIDS activity in general. Similar schemes – that extend this notion of celebrating a joint commitment – are in the process of being devised to meet a few other costs. Our constant endeavour is to mix and match the range of fund-raising mechanisms detailed above so as to ensure our financial sustainability.

SECTION TWO

HIV/AIDS Interventions at the Workplace

An Overview

There are several compelling arguments for focusing on HIV/AIDS interventions at the workplace. The one that is most frequently stressed in the international discourse is the potential of HIV/AIDS to debilitate the economy. The International Labour Organisation (ILO) warns that since HIV/AIDS hits hardest at the economically and sexually active population in the age group of 15 years and above, revenue loss due to absenteeism and time spent on training new workers to replace the loss of a skilled labour force, and labour shortage and increased cost of labour due to AIDS-related deaths, could together be severely damaging to the economy. Nowhere are the macro economic losses more glaring than in the African countries where one of the direct impacts of HIV infection is the 50 per cent drop in industrial production levels. The ILO warns companies to consider the loss to themselves due to diversion of their resources to health care expenditure, as sickness episodes among workers escalate in the wake of HIV infection. It urges them to consider intervening, both in their own and in the social interest, to preempt such losses.

However, the above image of an economic doomsday scenario caused by a depleting population due to AIDS has not yet gripped Indian industrial circles. Industry, like the rest of society, is still reluctant to give up the denial mode, and continues to be mired in the notion of the unique vulnerability of marginal groups – sex workers, truck drivers, men who have sex with men, and *hijras* (transvestites), all swimming in the miasma of poverty – who figure in sensational media reports. The understanding that in India there are many bridges through which the virus crosses over to the general population – to wives and children of truck drivers, to the wives of male clients who visit sex workers, to the wives of married men who have sex with other men, and wives of well-off and poor male workers whose jobs require long periods of separation from their families – is not yet fully appreciated by industry. There is also a sense of complacency that HIV/AIDS can be kept at bay by simply preventing it from entering the factory gates through mandatory testing of all job applicants.

To the extent that public attention has been focused on HIV/AIDS in the workplace and related issues of employment, it has been in relation to the violation of human rights. Employers violate human rights when they arrange for HIV tests without the knowledge or informed consent of employees, when they fire employees who test positive, when they deny employment to qualified job seekers because medical examinations that included HIV testing without consent show them up as HIV positive, when they make public positive employees' HIV status with the attendant stigma in the work environment, or when they marginalise positive employees into jobs that do not match their skills leading to demoralisation and stigma.

The whole issue of human rights violations at the workplace arising out of the HIV status of employees is a complex and compelling one that needs to be addressed by both legal and non-legal instruments. Some of these dimensions are discussed in the chapter in this book that deals with legal approaches to HIV/AIDS. The HIV/AIDS epidemic has spawned several human rights advocacy initiatives worldwide that are working towards articulating humane and enabling laws and practices relating to HIV/AIDS that protect the health and employment rights of workers. In India, the thrust of these efforts is to safeguard the equal rights to employment guaranteed by the Constitution. In this section, the focus is on non-legal workplace-led approaches to creating a human rights sensitive environment. The workplace offers a huge opportunity for employers in general to prevent or minimise the effects of the AIDS epidemic through the provision of AIDS awareness and education at the workplace itself. A pre-requisite is employers' willingness to be prompted to confront and reexamine their own deep-seated prejudices, and to replace these with enlightened social attitudes and workplace guidelines. Ideally, non-legal approaches complement legal provisions that safeguard workers' rights.

Discussion and social research on HIV/AIDS have often pointed to the potential that schools and colleges have to raise AIDS awareness among adolescents through sex education and sexuality and life skills counselling. While not underplaying the critical period of adolescence in this regard, such a self awareness and empowerment process remains central to the individual's capacity to protect himself/ herself from HIV infection, whatever the stage in the life cycle. Yet virtually no attention has been paid to the adult context of work where a considerable proportion of the out-of-school population in the age group 15 to 49 years may be found at any point in time.

Like educational institutions, workplaces are institutional contexts where large and fairly stable concentrations of people form captive audiences for health education. Educational programmes to raise awareness about HIV/AIDS prevention and management – and, indeed about health at any level – are most effective when they are carried out in a face-to-face and ongoing manner. They can make an optimal impact – be absorbed and retained – only when done sequentially, i.e., when they take the audience through various levels of understanding, from the simple to the more complex, best done when the audience is a reasonably stable one as compared with the one-off or sporadic contact that mass media 'messages' afford. Further, for awareness-raising to lead to positive and considered action on the part of the individual, it needs to be an iterative process, i.e., linked with periodic counselling within a trusted space which, in turn, may become a spur to voluntary check-up/testing and treatment.

Another factor that enhances the value of interventions at the workplace is the range of populations that may be found there. Close to 40 per cent of the total Indian population is in the workforce, of which around 60 per cent are involved in agriculture. This still leaves a sizeable workforce in urban occupations. In India, despite labour laws to the contrary, many workplace settings particularly in the unorganised sector also include non-adults, i.e., children or adolescents who work alongside adults and who come into contact with adults in unprotected adult-dominated environments, in the sense of exposure to sexual abuse (transport and hotel sectors, small scale industries that work in a putting-out system, to name just a few). It is now common wisdom that young people are among the most vulnerable to HIV/AIDS because they have little access to accurate knowledge about sex and sexuality, sources of infection or means of self-protection, besides being disadvantaged in terms of power equations vis-à-vis adults in work situations where their own economic vulnerability is high. AIDS awareness efforts by employers in such work environments can reach out to young people who are not in school or college.

Again, a number of modern industries (e.g., in the export sector, fisheries, garments, etc.) have a youthful, often unmarried, and predominantly female workforce. A number of these young women may be migrants, seeking to support themselves and their families back home. Like adolescents, they are among the most vulnerable in the HIV/AIDS epidemic. They may be prey to sexual exploitation at the workplace by powerful males who control their employment prospects (e.g. factory supervisors, contractors hiring labour gangs). At worst, their sexual exploitation may lead to spurious marriages that result in desertion, or in their being sold off, lured into or driven into prostitution. Reaching them in their workplaces could become an important route to get protective information across to them and teach them skills of negotiation. It would also demonstrate industry's commitment to the democratic values of the larger society, i.e., gender justice and access to knowledge as an empowering process.

A variety of studies have found that transmission of HIV infection happens most in environments where men are separated from their families. Migrant labour constitutes a high proportion of the working force in the country. Risky behaviour – purchasing commercial sex – by men is much higher when they are living away from their wives than when they have easy access to spousal sex. Once infected, these workers infect their unsuspecting wives when they go home on vacation or for agricultural operations. Uneven development across regions of the country makes for a significant migration of population to where the employment opportunities are; this may be from rural to urban, urban to urban or rural to rural areas, intra-state, inter-state and international. Men's general lack of awareness of the dangers of unprotected sex and their resort to commercial sex make marriage the greatest risk factor for the women who are their current or potential wives, and through them for their children. In jobs that require considerable geographical and social mobility, the relative isolation from the family combined with long working hours may lead men into casual sexual relationships and render them highly vulnerable to STDs/HIV/AIDS. This applies not only to poor migrant labour but equally to those in better paying and skilled jobs, older and generally married men, as found by some recent ILO and UNDP studies of industrial labour in Chennai. All these aspects present an unusual challenge of HIV infection spreading through various routes, along with which comes its long period of invisibility, and subsequent manifestation through opportunistic infections.

Due to the many sensitive sexual and socio-political issues relating to AIDS, teaching by peer educators and collective learning by peers has become an established mechanism for creating a climate of opinion in support of responsible sexual behaviour and dispelling misconceptions. Like the school/educational setting, the workplace provides a potentially 'safe' yet powerful place for dealing with people's attitudes, values and sexual behaviour. This is because, despite their varied personal backgrounds, people who share a workplace (even if only as contract labour for certain periods of time), i.e., a common way of earning a living, share a familiar social space for interaction, gossip, exchange of information and experiences, and for influencing one another's opinions and behaviour, not just relating to the job, but also outside of it. While the sense of community may be stronger in some settings than in others, it exists in some form in all workplaces. Influential members within these groups can exert positive influence on others.

There are other reasons as well why workplaces are safe environments for imparting AIDS education. Unlike most other communicable diseases where transmission is by air, water or food, thus having the potential to infect many more people and therefore more difficult to control, HIV/AIDS is transmitted only by sexual and blood contact which does not as a rule happen in workplaces, other than accidental injuries within healthcare settings where transmission can be controlled through adoption of universal precautions and post-exposure prophylaxis (PEP). Hence, the workplace also offers an excellent base for education into how HIV is not transmitted; this is equally important and can contribute much to removing fear and prejudice. Since transmission in the course of casual everyday contact in the work environment is extremely rare, AIDS education could remove fears of working alongside infected colleagues by emphasising that the implements and articles of everyday use do not act as reservoirs for the virus. Information dissemination on nutrition and self-care can benefit not only HIV positive workers but others as well. The demonstration that positive persons can continue to work and lead useful lives further diminishes stigma. At the same time, by educating workers and management on simple and safe practices in order to prevent the possibility of contracting HIV infection, it can empower them to deal with HIV both in the workplace and outside without fear, prejudice or discrimination, rather than resort to unjust practices such as resenting the presence of HIV infected persons at the workplace, or shunning/ turning violent against them in the community of residence. AIDS education needs to be directed at all categories of employees and not confined to lower level staff alone, since prejudices and fears are deeply ingrained in all rungs of the class hierarchy. Nor must it unduly stress 'high risk' groups, and convey that only they are at risk, since in reality all are at risk.

Further, earning members of a family tend to be influential opinion makers within the family setting and can potentially carry back important health-related understanding from the workplace. In professions such as the army and the police force whose members tend to get exposed to a wide range of modernising influences, earning members have been important carriers of a wide variety of knowledge and practices for their families back home. The same ought to apply in the case of sensitively imparted AIDS education.

In terms of personal emotional tragedy, the possibility of economic losses to workers and their families due to sickness, resulting in indebtedness and total impoverishment, and the horrific possibility of whole families getting infected or parents leaving behind orphans, present huge challenges. The spread of the HIV/AIDS epidemic also holds out the possibility of losses to industry and, the forward and backward linkages of these with the widespread poverty and poor state of public health services in the country. One effective way of responding to these challenges is if private, public and NGO sectors come together to form partnerships. What follows is an account of how PREPARE – a development NGO – which was new to the field of HIV/AIDS and did not identify it as its core concern, nonetheless responded to the presence of HIV among its constituent populations with a workplace-based intervention programme. Applying its vision of development and gender justice to the area of AIDS prevention and building on its own organisational strengths, PREPARE was one of the earliest organisations in the country to innovate within the industrial environment. PREPARE works in Tamil Nadu and Andhra Pradesh – among the two hardest hit states in the country where the HIV epidemic is concerned – and in an industrial zone reputed to be the second largest concentration of industries in South and South East Asia. In the course of its attempts to build partnerships with industrial workers, trade unions, managements, industrial associations, Employees' State Insurance hospitals and workers' families and local communities, PREPARE found itself having to fight not only resistance to and stigmatisation of HIV concerns within industry, but also its own devaluation and stigmatisation by managements because its HIV/AIDS programme touched the taboo areas of sexuality and sexual behaviour. Not least was the challenge of coming to terms with reservations and inhibitions within the PREPARE team itself. The chapter candidly discusses the learning experience for all concerned.

Tackling HIV/AIDS in the Industrial Workforce

The Efforts of PREPARE

JUDE STEPHENS AND DAISY DHARMARAJ

PREPARE – an NGO working in the area of disaster preparedness and focusing on the rights of *dalits* (those who are lowest in the caste hierarchy), tribals and fisherfolk in Tamil Nadu and Andhra Pradesh – was set up in 1983 by a group of young professionals with backgrounds in medicine, engineering, social work, with the objective of promoting social, economic and political justice, environmental protection, food security, gender equity and human rights. Health was only one component in this broad developmental portfolio. The unanticipated emergence of HIV/AIDS among some sections of its constituent populations driven by poverty and seasonal migration, and the high levels of sickness and premature deaths that came in its wake, propelled PREPARE to consider extending its work into HIV/AIDS. One of PREPARE's HIV/AIDS programmes soon came to encompass urban and highway based sex workers, truckers, urban slum populations and street children, and factory workers in an industrial belt close to the city of Chennai in Tamil Nadu.

PREPARE's office is located in the heart of the Ambattur Industrial Estate in west Chennai, Tamil Nadu, and this had a major role in the decision to launch an intervention among factory workers. In 1996, when PREPARE first began this intervention, there were no precedents for it to go by. Despite the well-known epidemiological fact that in India over 85 per cent of all reported cases of HIV belong to the sexually active and economically productive age group, the industrial workforce – among the most easily accessible sections of this age group – was (and is so even today) largely ignored in HIV/AIDS prevention and education programmes in the country. With virtually no road map to follow, PREPARE found itself having to innovate within an indifferent if not outrightly hostile environment for the reception of ideas regarding sexual behaviour, sexually transmitted infections, and condom use – all taboo areas – seen by employers to have no consequence for the industrial environment of work, productivity and profits. Working doggedly, and alternating its strategies between workers, senior and middle managements, business and trade associations, older and younger employees, men and women workers, board rooms, factory gates, the Employees State Insurance hospitals and working class housing colonies, PREPARE was able to slowly create a space for serious examination by all these actors of the links between personal behaviour and social outcomes.

Framing the issue

Ambattur Industrial Estate is South East Asia's second largest industrial unit. There are now between 2,000 official and 1,000 unofficial industrial units in the Ambattur/Padi area and about 200,000 to 300,000 people who work in these units. Of these, 40 per cent are women due to the existence of a large number of export-oriented garment industries that prefer to employ women. The conditions under which these women – and particularly the young girls among them – work make them vulnerable to HIV/AIDS. Generally, the existence of a sizeable sexually active population, and the fact that many of them – both women and men – are migrants living alone away from families and exposed to casual sex and associated high risk situations, added to the significance of this industrial workforce for the purpose of our intervention.

Migrant girls come to work in the industries from towns and cities as near as 70-80 kilometres, and from villages as far as 1,000-1,500 kilometres away. Some are run-away girls while others have come with the consent of their families. They live either in groups renting a house or in hostels. Many try and stay away from relationships until their families get them married; some strike up acquaintances/friendships with men whom they come in contact with, but may or may not marry them. All the supervisors in these units are male. Supervisors are required to certify the products made by the women before the latter get paid, and the price for this is often sexual favours. Although not on an organised basis, this harassment tends to be common. The economic and sexual exploitation of the women at the workplace by male supervisors, whom they have to please in order to save themselves from being retrenched is another contributing factor to a high-risk situation. Gender concerns and sexual exploitation are, therefore, intrinsic to any intervention in such a work environment.

The objectives of the project thus came to be formulated as follows:

1. to sensitise the workforce to a basic understanding of STDs/HIV/AIDS and issues related to alcohol, drugs, sexuality, power and gender relations;
2. to enhance STDs/HIV/AIDS prevention by promoting the use of condoms and providing information about its proper use in STDs/RTIs care; and
3. to develop an AIDS policy in the workplace that opposes discrimination in keeping with the guidelines laid out by the International Labour Organisation and the World Health Organisation (ILO/WHO).

Initiating the intervention

We began by profiling the local industrial scene: the sectoral spread, size of firms in terms of both magnitude of capital and number of persons employed, recruitment patterns, facilities and other non-wage benefits offered to employees, employer-employee relationships and, business associations and trade unions. This was followed by a field survey with a sample size of 50 women and 200 men employees as a basis for designing the proposed health education intervention. The survey threw up many misconceptions and prejudices, notably: that HIV infected persons should be shunned, that HIV/AIDS is curable if detected early, that women are the prime cause for the spread of HIV/AIDS, that HIV/AIDS can be spread through sharing toilets and food, and that persons affected by HIV/AIDS can be easily recognised by their external appearance. Our conclusion was that employees in general were negative in their attitudes towards HIV/AIDS. There was an attitude of fear and stigma regarding STDs and AIDS, and of refusal to work with HIV positive co-workers or claim for rights to a disease-free environment.

And what of the employers? Our next step was to create awareness among the managements about the need for an HIV/AIDS prevention programme in the workplace. We met with company heads on an individual basis, discussed our mission to offer health education to their employees, and requested for the opportunity to put this into effect. We stressed the socio-economic impact that HIV/AIDS would have on companies if they did not take preventive efforts now: the loss of trained human resources; number of days lost due to sick leave; reduction in productivity; replacement and retraining costs when positive workers became totally disabled; medical costs; insurance costs; costs of litigation if managements demanded the resignation of infected persons; animosity of uninformed/misinformed colleagues demanding discrimination against infected persons; loss of morale among the worker community when loved ones passed away; and, discrimination against working women.

Our starting assumption had been that data on HIV/AIDS prevalence and epidemiology would be sufficient to persuade companies to adopt a prevention programme. But we were wrong; managements did not believe that HIV/AIDS had reached the factory gates. What they 'saw' was plenty of publicity on the television, newspapers and radio, and they believed that employees must surely be picking up all there was to know about HIV/AIDS. They were complacent that even if their own workforce were to get infected, the numbers would be small enough for them to manage the situation; if necessary, they could even prevent HIV/AIDS entering the factory through pre-employment screening of new employees.

Although reluctant to give us time for our educational programme during working hours, most company heads were willing to allow us at least about half-an-hour with their employees during the lunch break. They also permitted us to meet with their workers after factory working hours. These concessions, although small, helped us flag off our work. Initially, our effort was limited to establishing rapport with the workers during the short work breaks. Wherever we encountered interest, we continued the conversations after factory hours, often accompanying the workers to the bus stops outside the factory from where they left for their homes. Gradually, we progressed to conducting small group meetings within the factory premises in the evenings.

The protocols

These random informal meetings prepared the ground for a more structured educational intervention and campaign. At the core of this was intensive discussion. After an initial discussion laying out the basic facts about HIV/AIDS, the interaction moved to a higher level of complexity. The course that we designed consisted of around eight modules of one hour each, catering to 30 to 40 participants at a time. The modules offered comprehensive information about the following: the nature of HIV infection, its relationship with STDs, safer sex methods, the need for a collective/community response to HIV/AIDS, responsible individual behaviour, positive attitude towards those infected, counselling and testing aspects, gender aspects, and issues of ethics, human rights and legal obligations.

We chose a variety of tools for awareness-creation and education, which we pilot-tested and refined to suit our audience.

Slides and an overhead projector were used to explain the basic nature of HIV infection. Video shows provided a comprehensive picture of the progression from HIV to AIDS and the complications that could arise along the way. Flash cards and flip charts served to promote knowledge on sexually transmitted diseases (STDs), reproductive tract infections (RTIs) and HIV/AIDS. Condom demonstrations were done using bananas and candles. We also presented some case histories – with the active involvement of known HIV positive volunteers – to explain risks, fears and attitudes. Finally, we used group discussions and games to focus on collective and/or individual responsibility, encourage non-judgemental attitudes and personalise the issue of HIV/AIDS.

The factual slide and video shows proved to be the most effective educational tools, laying the ground in a non-personal way for what came later, i.e., the group discussions and case histories that elicited the emotional involvement of the participants. Girls in the age group of 16-20 were worried about vaginal infections, menstrual problems, pregnancy, sexuality and gender concerns, and about how they could escape from high-risk situations. They also sought more knowledge about symptoms and signs of HIV and about its cure. Among married women, the dominant concerns were STDs and RTIs, communicability of these conditions, risks associated with multi-partner sex, condom usage, HIV/AIDS symptoms and complications, breast-feeding by HIV positive women, and cure of HIV/AIDS.

Interesting methodological insights emerged from the group discussions, pertaining mainly to group composition. Heterogeneous groups – whether gender mixed or combining different ages or of mixed marital status – were not successful in eliciting meaningful participation. Sexuality could not be openly discussed in any of the groups, and married men and women tended to reflect the most conservative opinions and to be the most judgemental and less open to change than unmarried persons. Younger workers proved to be much less inhibited generally and more able to identify with our own team members most of whom were also young, resulting in a more frank discussion on sexuality among these participants. However, even among the young we found that sexuality is not a topic that is discussed at all, even among close friends.

While it was not easy to totally reformulate the health education materials to individually cater to each kind of group, we learnt to use the same materials differently each time. Our interventions seemed to act as a catalyst to opening up communication, and we could only hope that this was the beginning of a process that would help prevent gender exploitation and STDs in the future. We realised that it would have been valuable to enact high-risk situations or present them through videos in order to bring hidden concerns out into the open, at least within small groups. Despite the constraints arising out of the heterogeneous composition of groups, this broader interaction helped us identify smaller groups for further discussion. We were also able to convey our openness to meeting people on a one-on-one basis, and for informal counselling sessions either within the company premises or near the bus stops. Sessions held at the end of the working day proved to be more relaxed and open than those held during breaks in work, and we tried to take advantage of this. Another constraint on free interaction during work breaks was the occasional presence of management representatives, which seemed to act as a dampener.

The roadblocks

There were several obstacles that came in the way of making substantive progress with the workers' education. A large proportion of the workers at this industrial estate live at a considerable distance away and are anxious to get back to their homes and hostels early. Some have to travel for an hour or an hour and a half by train each way to do so. It was hard to convince them to stay on after factory hours for the discussions and counselling sessions that we were organising for them. There were occasions when only two or at most five persons would turn up for a discussion meeting.

Comprehending the connection between sexual pleasure and incurable infection and eventual death proved to be a difficult task for them. While sexually transmitted infection was a reality experienced by at least some, HIV/AIDS was still an unfamiliar phenomenon to all. None among them had seen a death due to AIDS. When conducting awareness sessions in the factory premises within the constraints of time and space, we were unable to segregate the younger from the older workers, and this had its own implications for the effectiveness of discussions relating to sexuality or STDs/HIV/AIDS. Older married male workers found it embarrassing to talk openly about sex in a group situation where young people were also present. In turn, their attitudes dampened the enthusiasm and humour of young males in particular when the latter tried to swap stories about sexual escapades. Unwillingness of one age group to look at pictures of STDs in the presence of the other age group was another instance of mutual inhibition.

Another fact that they found hard to come to terms with was that there was no cure for HIV/AIDS. Among this section of people, Western medical information is not always accepted as the truth, and nor are statistics seen to be proving that most HIV positive persons suffer and eventually die. In a culture where a multitude of traditional healthcare systems abound, just about everybody has an opinion on the efficacy of one or other system. We found it difficult to convince the workers that AIDS had no cure in any known system of medicine. Adding to our difficulty was the fact that every now and again some publication would carry a story about a drug trial being conducted by some alternative health care system. Again, news magazines commonly read by the workers often reported quacks making unethical claims about wonder cures. We realised that we would need great patience to deal with this.

Although women were able to see the rationale of condom usage, they felt that they were not in control, that men wielded more power within the relationship, and that women did not have any bargaining power, especially within marriage. This opened up issues of gender relations and power, but it was not easy to hold protracted discussions for want of time.

Our original rosy plan had been to craft a three party coalition consisting of PREPARE, managements and workers. Initially, the managements of the factories that we approached treated us with some cordiality, but after a couple of meetings they began proving elusive. Further moves by us met with apathy and, on occasion, even passive resistance. They clearly showed no eagerness to involve themselves in the cause of HIV/AIDS.

Frustrated, we turned to the trade unions. In our advocacy attempts with them, we focused on the rights of employees – rights to information, to choose whether to be screened or not for STDs and HIV, and to confidentiality – and on how these rights could be violated when HIV/AIDS entered the industrial sector in a significant way. We stressed the need to look at HIV/AIDS as just another chronic disease, the long-duration treatment that it entailed, and issues of insurance and management share of responsibility in meeting the costs of treatment and care, similar to the case of any other chronic disease. We emphasised management responsibilities in the provision of universal protection methods in case of accidents and in treatment centres, in facilitating condom availability, and in dealing with issues of discrimination and retrenchment of those infected.

At this point the personnel department called us in for a discussion as a prelude to granting official permission to mount an intervention. Several factors seemed to have been contributing to their general initial hesitancy to allow discussion of anything related to sex within the factory premises; there was a fear of being seen by the workers to be condoning promiscuity, and an apprehension that an easy familiarity might get established if such discussions took place in their presence. Seeing the ease with which we handled the whole aspect of sexuality in our health education sessions, they were now feeling somewhat encouraged.

The new bend in the road

We were beginning to realise that for our programme to be successful and sustainable it had to be much more flexible, innovative and inclusive. The challenge was to come up with interventions that were acceptable to both managements and employees. We needed to persuade managements to adopt a worker-friendly approach with regard to HIV/AIDS. And our work with employees had to build-in peer influence in the direction of safer sex. Initially at least, our follow-up interaction with employees would need to remain outside of the factory gates. As outsiders, our own approach within the factory would need to be one of keeping a low profile and remaining unobtrusive, all the while taking care to steer clear of controversial or bipartisan issues, particularly those touching on management-trade union relations.

As a first step, we formed an advisory committee consisting of representatives of NGOs, lawyers, trade unions, business, management, specialists in sexual health and communication and counsellors, to help steer our project performance. We classified the companies in the industrial estate into three groups: those that were not favourable to HIV/AIDS intervention within company premises; those which gave us space to interact with employees within a restricted time frame; and those which valued our intervention and facilitated it willingly.

With the first group our strategy was to work through the trade/management Associations. It is these Associations that discuss and decide on larger issues, and lobby in the external environment for benefits to their trade/industry. We held discussions individually and in groups with members of the Boards of these Associations where we spoke of our mission of making workers aware of HIV/AIDS and means for its prevention and control, and highlighted why open discussions on sexuality were a basic requirement for this. What had particular impact was our presentation of the global comparative picture of why many leading industries both in industrialised and developing countries had formulated HIV/AIDS prevention policies focusing on their workforces, particularly the progressive steps taken by industrial organisations and governments of countries such as Canada, Zimbabwe and Uganda to combat the threat of HIV/AIDS. We also spoke of the ILO convention on the subject, and the recognition by our own Confederation of Indian Industry (CII) of the need for HIV/AIDS education in the workplace. Our presentations of case histories relating to employees, housewives and children evoked particular interest. We were gradually able to leverage the Associations to let us hold sensitisation workshops along the same lines for the managements of their member companies.

In time, we were able to witness a remarkable change in attitudes, particularly among the large industries, as the understanding grew that HIV/AIDS could be a threat to the prosperity of their businesses and also something that could disrupt their own lives and those of their loved ones. This had a demonstration effect on the smaller industries that now also started opening their doors to us. We began to strategically receive requests to organise health camps for employees. The health camps that we organised included screening for diabetes, hypertension, tuberculosis, STDs and skin infections, as well as obstetric and gynaecological examinations and advice for women. A central element in every camp was an attractively designed stall on STDs and HIV/AIDS, equipped with different kinds of audio-visual aids and condom demonstrations. In rooms specially set aside for the purpose, sexual health counsellors were at hand for confidential consultations and to answer queries. We were able to reach many workers with information on HIV/AIDS, and persons with a history of unprotected sex were screened for STDs at their request. However, we ensured that no HIV testing was done, although the managements concerned were keen that we do so. Young girls with STDs and RTIs found these camps particularly useful as they were able to access sensitive and professional care as well as counselling with regard to safer sex, early and complete treatment of STDs, and partner treatment.

We also established an association with the Employees State Insurance (ESI) hospitals. These are the official agencies that address the health concerns of industrial workers. They are closely tied with provision of reimbursement of medical expenses, medical certification, insurance and accident schemes, as well as retirement benefits. Fortunately, the medical officers in these hospitals were sympathetic to our concerns. We held exhibitions in these hospitals, and conducted workshops and counselling sessions.

Both the health camps and the hospital-based programmes helped increase acceptance of our intervention by the industries. On average, on an annual basis, we covered around 120 industrial units, and held over 200 sensitisation workshops separately for male workers, women workers, young canteen boys, workers' wives and workers' families, covering in all about 1,600 men and 900 women. We also operated a dedicated medical clinic for unmarried and married women workers of a cluster of garment industries, with a lady doctor in attendance for STDs/RTIs and general gynaecological screening and treatment.

However, we cannot claim that our efforts have led to significant proactive measures on the part of industry either in relation to prevention and control of HIV/AIDS among their workforce, or to enhanced respect for the human rights of HIV positive persons. What we have been able to observe is a certain measure of restraint in the matter of retrenchment of those found to be infected, and in carrying out compulsory pre-employment HIV testing of prospective employees. Some employers continue to make VDRL/HIV testing of provisionally selected employees mandatory, with or without their knowledge, as part of the selection process and in case of training or promotion schemes for existing employees. We have not been able to make a significant dent on the long-standing feeling among such employers that they have the right to conduct mandatory medical examinations in order to protect themselves from low productivity and medical expenses that may ensue if unhealthy employees are selected. Any employee challenging such examination or blood test could be refused employment on some other pretext, or subjected to disciplinary action on grounds of insubordination. The HIV antibody testing, as a method of screening individuals, is not always done correctly. Nor is it accompanied by the mandatory confidential pre- and post-test counselling. In the manner in which it is done, it violates the basic individual right to privacy and dignity. We continued to lobby with the managements on this issue. After about three years of such efforts we have been able to bring about a change in their attitude.

Despite these successes, however, it was our conviction that our main thrust ought to continue to be in the direction of strengthening our fellowship with the workers in the industrial belt. Within the factories, we worked with Worker Education Groups (WEGs). Every industrial establishment has a WEG comprising representatives of workers hand-picked by the management. Seniority of service, level of skill and work performance are the main criteria for nomination to the WEG. The objective behind industries setting up the WEGs is to have a cadre of workers who can act as peer educators for dissemination of skills required for newer methods and technologies of production. We trained the WEGs to act as peer educators for raising awareness about HIV/AIDS, risk factors, prevention, control and behaviour change, human rights and gender dimensions.

Simultaneously, we intensified our interaction with the workers outside of factory premises. We put up tents and exhibitions along the main thoroughfares where we held video shows, street plays and magic shows that conveyed STD and HIV/AIDS messages in entertaining ways. We made ourselves visibly available for quality interaction and for counselling. We started a bi-monthly newsletter for wide circulation, called SAVAAL ("Poser" or "Challenge") in Tamil and English, containing brief and clear messages. Within and outside factory premises we put up HIV/AIDS prevention messages in order to reinforce our other efforts, and held periodical health camps focusing on STD/RTI care within the factories. During festivals and associated celebrations organised by companies and in the colonies where employees live with their families, we organised street plays and cultural shows. For the younger women who dominate the employee profile of the garment making units, we ran regular sexual health and hygiene workshops, talks and counselling sessions. We began a telephone help line to further supplement these efforts. We also involved other local NGOs, medical institutions and community workers in our awareness campaigns, and they became valuable resources for our health camps organised specially for garment industry workers. We also attempted to promote condom use through conventional outlets such as medical and general provision stores, and through non-conventional outlets within company settings such as vending machines placed in toilets and within departments.

We soon extended our campaign to cover the entire network of people whom factory workers relate to on a day-to-day basis outside of the workplace. We began with barbers, whom we saw as people with strong potential to influence off-workplace behaviour. The barbers in the area have a well-knit network, and we used their saloons to our advantage as dispensing outlets for awareness-raising calendars, pamphlets and signboards with AIDS messages and condoms. We did the same with teashop operators, wine shop and petrol (gasoline) station owners and chemists. At a few selected petrol (gasoline) stations equipped with large-scale departmental stores and retiring rooms for use by consumers, we placed condom dispensing machines; the condoms were replaced fortnightly and their distribution audited. The drivers of auto rickshaws – a popular three-wheeler mode of transport – were an important 'high risk' audience for our efforts. Like truck drivers on national highways, auto rickshaw drivers plying the streets of the city and suburbs come into easy contact with sex workers. They also identify and ferry clients – and these are often factory employees – to sex workers. We trained them to be peer educators, to prominently display HIV/AIDS prevention messages on their vehicles, and to distribute prevention education materials to passengers, particularly those visiting sex workers. We also organised camps on the subject of STDs at the three main auto rickshaw stands in the industrial area, and encouraged drivers to refer known customers to us for counselling and treatment.

By now HIV testing was generally on the increase in the area, most of it involuntary, and this was becoming an instrument to identify and discriminate against persons found to be positive. Hospitals were conducting tests on those coming in for admission as in-patients, and refusing those testing positive.

General practitioners and companies were also testing people without their knowledge, and the results – if positive – were being used to either deny employment after interviews or to terminate employment. None of those being tested was receiving any counselling, either pre-test or post-test. We identified 52 laboratory technicians in the area for training in the clinical and ethical aspects of HIV/AIDS, and encouraged them to refer their clients to us for counselling.

We also followed up the workers' health camps in other ways. Those who had tested VDRL positive were visited by PREPARE programme staff in their homes, counselled and motivated for treatment. This included those residing in nearby towns and villages. PREPARE programme staff escorted them to local ESI or government hospitals where they supervised their treatment. This outreach service also included the wives of these workers. With them our focus was on teaching the importance of consistent and proper condom use.

Street theatre – conducted by a professional street theatre group that worked with us – was an important instrument in our mass-education campaigns. We identified 18 colonies in this industrial belt where we held regular street plays. These were strategic locations where workers hung out after working hours, shopping, drinking tea or waiting for their buses. Many women, too, gathered to watch them. The street plays were well received. The basic objective of the plays was to make people comfortable with the issue of STD/HIV/AIDS. They carried messages about STDs, condom use, HIV/AIDS and the importance of showing compassion to those infected and affected.

Looking back, looking forward

Over the years, both workers and managements have by and large opened up to discussing the AIDS threat. This is a big change from the earlier apathy and misconceptions and fears. Nor is HIV/AIDS any longer a distant threat as more and more persons test positive every day. It is a measure of some satisfaction that we have turned a corner with many of the managements/owners of the industrial units in the area. As a far cry from the passive resistance that we faced in the initial period of our intervention, some companies are now actually meeting our programme costs. There are, however, several others that continue to be in a state of denial with regard to HIV/AIDS.

Our scheme of placing condoms in toilets and departments in factories floundered. Although we thought we had overcome the initial hesitation among company heads who feared misuse and protests from workers and possible labour problems, particularly in the garment industries where women and men work together and where owners and managements both feared that it might be construed as a sanction to promiscuity, we were unable to make headway. We shifted to entrusting the WEGs, personnel officers and occupational health staff – the last-mentioned were a feature particularly of large-scale industrial units – with the task of condom distribution. We informed the workers about this arrangement and monitored its functioning, making regular visits to receive feedback and replenish stocks. Through sustained sensitisation, we were able to slowly erode the stigma relating to condoms. The approach succeeded wherever it was supported by the presence of friendly and informal personnel/social officers or occupational health staff. However, officials who distanced themselves from workers were not the only obstacles to sustaining this process. Where we worked with WEGs, their tenure was too brief to allow much progress; every year new representatives were appointed to the Groups, and PREPARE programme staff had to conduct sensitisation sessions all over again for the new incumbents.

Working with the Employees State Insurance (ESI) staff was particularly rewarding. Industrial workers and their spouses visiting ESI dispensaries proved to be a captive audience for condom education and promotion. We were able to counsel those diagnosed with STDs or RTIs how to use the condoms supplied by us. We were gratified to gradually observe that those who had become familiar with condom usage were using it as a preventive method, and particularly so in high-risk situations. We also found the ESI authorities open to discussing issues pertaining to medical management of workers with HIV/AIDS. We were also able to broach issues of provisions relating to funeral expenses, care and support to the terminally ill, and supportive ethics in terms of recommending insurance, leave and other benefits to affected employees. All this makes us optimistic about the prospect of 'AIDS friendly' ESI policies, given sufficient ground work, support from sympathetic NGOs and political will.

Our experience with workers has taught us that constant reinforcement of awareness is necessary. Workers – like everybody else – are liable to not give importance to what they have learnt. What is required is a work plan that reminds them from time to time about the presence of STDs/HIV/AIDS in their midst and the need for their active role in self-protection. Accordingly, we modified our bi-monthly newsletter SAVAAL to a simple monthly leaflet with illustrations and messages targeting the message of STDs/HIV/AIDS. These illustrations are prominently displayed on company and departmental notice boards. The initiative has borne fruit; it has enabled us to further reinforce messages, facilitate referrals and enhance the response to our telephone counselling service. A number of workers now come to us for counselling on their own initiative, and women are far more proactive than men in their interactions with us.

We have continued to contribute to building the skills and capacities of the community-based organisations (CBOs) in the area through information sharing, distribution of educational materials and training. We also work with a network of NGOs in Chennai city and its environs working on prevention of HIV/AIDS among sex workers and their clients. The training that we impart to all these groups relate to: programme implementation of HIV/AIDS-related projects, such as needs assessment, building on objectives and activities, programme planning and review; guidance on setting quantitative and qualitative parameters/targets for monitoring and evaluating HIV/AIDS work; condom programming; and building HIV/AIDS prevention into developmental initiatives. We also relate to a range of NGOs and positive people's groups in Tamil Nadu as sounding boards for our project plans.

Introspection

As an organisation with the mission of working for development, health has been an important area of work for PREPARE since its inception. Three principles have guided us in this priority. Health is a felt need of disadvantaged communities; therefore, a new group wishing to work with such communities can gain access and acceptability through health interventions. Although it is the responsibility to the State to meet the health needs of people, health interventions help raise awareness and empower people, thus acting as powerful tools of health advocacy towards obtaining health rights. Finally, health is a good indicator of the socio-economic well-being of a community and leads the intervening team into areas of basic and crucial needs, enabling them to address these needs on a priority basis. When HIV/AIDS first appeared in the country, it did not seem to us to conform to this holistic view of health in relation to development. Slides were being flashed on the causes and effects, condoms were being advocated as the sole saving factor, and HIV/AIDS itself was being projected as a medical problem requiring a vertical approach, rather than as a social and economic problem requiring multi-pronged approaches including individual and community-level decision-making. The question before us was whether we as a development organisation had any role to play in relation to this disease and, if so, how. We thrashed this out within PREPARE, and the consensus at the time was that HIV/AIDS was not our priority and was best left to the health sector.

At this juncture, HIV infection surfaced among the migrant fisherfolk in Nellore-Prakasam districts of Andhra Pradesh with whom PREPARE was working at the time. Suddenly, several men in our communities were dying. Our examination of the problem revealed stark connections between HIV/AIDS and the acute poverty and helplessness among the people we were addressing: *dalits*, fisher folk and tribals and particularly their women. The more we probed, the clearer it became to us that HIV/AIDS was a disease contracted by people who had no access to information, who had to leave their families to migrate seasonally in search of employment, and by girls who had to resort to prostitution in order to feed themselves, collect money for their own marriage, and who could never free themselves from sexual and economic exploitation by men, rendering them highly vulnerable to HIV/AIDS. It was this conviction that HIV/AIDS is a developmental problem and a problem of gender injustice, and that our substantial experience in dealing with socio-economic and political problems gave us a meaningful role to play that finally propelled PREPARE to enter the HIV/AIDS field in the interests of these marginalised populations.

Initially, we familiarised ourselves with the medical aspects of HIV – the causative organism, the disease process, diagnosis, counselling, and prevention by safe sex – all of which were easy to learn and also non-controversial. Literature on these aspects was available in plenty, and we used the global literature to broaden our perspective. The experience of African countries was particularly helpful in this regard, even though they seemed to be following what we saw as an essentially Western approach. We also documented the available information and experiences of NGOs both within and outside India. We began designing our intervention using some of the available slides, but were soon developing new ones. The major communication problems with using the existing materials for our rural and illiterate communities were their strict use of medical terms, and the cultural and linguistic unfamiliarity of what the materials were conveying. We therefore developed our own role-plays and charts in settings that were familiar without, for example, the alien cartoon figures or virus pictures.

Our awareness campaign was just getting underway when a horrific incident took place in a village near Chikaluripet in Andhra Pradesh that received wide media coverage. A man had died of AIDS, and his wife who was a sex worker was burnt alive by a local mob. Our project team in Andhra Pradesh visited the area. Even though the atmosphere was charged, we decided to hold discussions with community leaders to seek their cooperation in starting HIV/AIDS educational work. We set up an exhibition of charts, pictures and slide shows followed by discussions with the local population. It was in the course of this that we learnt that the Guntur-Prakasam highway in the vicinity had a high concentration of sex workers, and that Chikaluripet was a major red light area. We adopted the whole area for intensive HIV/AIDS related work, due to its strategic importance as a focal point for the spread of HIV/AIDS. Thus began our involvement with sex workers who operated along the highway. To our surprise, there was no evidence of monetary or material comfort in their lives, something that is supposed to accrue from what is often seen as the high income earning potential of the sex trade. What we found instead were highly exploited and/or poverty-stricken women; some were in the grip of local mafia and politicians, and most had no life of their own. While others manipulated them for their own ends, they themselves were the objects of public revulsion. Although our first instinct was to condemn such an exploitative system, we thought it strategic to build an amicable relationship with the brokers, pimps and madams who were controlling these women so as to gain access to the sex workers.

The intervention among fisherfolk and sex workers was the PREPARE team's first experience of openly discussing issues relating to sexuality. It did not prove easy. With most of the team consisting of young unmarried persons – women and men – from conservative rural backgrounds, the dominant feeling was that it was culturally inappropriate to explicitly discuss sexuality, whether within the team or with communities outside. There was discomfort also with the idea of accepting sex work as normal or justifiable, or that people could choose to have different sexual orientations. However, if we had to engage in HIV/AIDS-related work we had to develop the ability to handle the topic of sexuality in ways that reached everyone in the community, earned their confidence and, in time, influenced their sexual behaviour.

The fact that one of us – Daisy, the head of the PREPARE team and a medical doctor – was always present as part of the team, particularly during the rapport-building phase of work with each population group and regularly throughout the interventions, helped make the younger team members feel supported although it did not lessen the challenge for them. They grew in maturity and experience as they learnt to face each situation. Again, although we spoke of the need for empathy with infected persons and those living with AIDS, there apparently was a hesitation among team members to sit with positive people, eat with them, hold their hand, or hug them in support. When I as team leader did all these spontaneously, it was easier for the team to follow suit, as they themselves confessed later. Even for me, it was quite a challenge and experience to be standing at *dhabas* (food stalls) on the highway in the middle of the night along with my team of boys, waiting for trucks to stop by, and then engaging in discussions lasting into the small hours of the morning with truckers – and often sex workers – about sex and HIV, and teaching them about condom use. In a scenario where the only other women on the streets at that hour were sex workers, my presence made an impact on the *dhaba* owners and truckers about PREPARE's seriousness and commitment to addressing the problem of HIV/AIDS.

As we worked on the highways at night talking to sex workers and truckers, we often had run-ins with the police who would stop and interrogate us. Sometimes I was the lone woman in the team, particularly in circumstances where the younger women members found it difficult to participate. Displaying great insensitivity and prejudice the police would accuse us of encouraging prostitution, brand us as clients, and insist that we were carrying pornographic literature. These were embarrassing and sensitive moments for the young members of the team, as well as for their family members who nevertheless steadfastly stood by them in their work. We had to repeatedly confront police officials and convince them of our work; two strategies that proved helpful were inviting them to officiate at our public functions in order to expose them to our interventions, and issuing identity cards to our own members.

At the time that our team of young men and women began work in the industrial belt, other problems surfaced. When the young women engaged male workers in discussion, the men would either not meet their eyes or, at the other extreme, try to make advances. My own background (and therefore 'authority') as a doctor eased our acceptance in the industrial area, but it did not spare me from deliberate attempts to embarrass me. For instance, I would be asked unnecessarily elaborate questions on different forms of sexual behaviour. It was obvious to the team that all the women members faced this disadvantage vis-à-vis the men we encountered, and it created a bond of solidarity amongst us, and encouraged us to face challenges and see how we could overcome them in a professional manner.

In HIV education, generally, the Western approach prevails. Permissiveness – or the possibility of multi-partner sex – is an underlying concept, and acceptance of it the main tool to deal with the topic of safe sex. A judgemental approach is discouraged as it is seen to inhibit people – and particularly the young – from opening up, thereby making it difficult to assess their behaviour and, therefore, their vulnerability. This approach was and still is a major mental block for some of us in PREPARE and difficult to come to terms with. It is our belief that HIV/AIDS might have been first analysed in the context of Western society, but this does not preclude the fact that non-Western communities have their own religious and cultural norms and forms of social control which need to be respected and taken as starting points for any intervention in their midst. While maintaining a non-judgemental attitude in relation to persons who practise multi-partner sex or 'non-conventional' forms of sexual behaviour, and having full respect for the individual in person-to-person contacts, our position remains one of advocating faithfulness to one partner. This includes homosexual relationships. We maintain that Indian society does not require going through a sexual revolution or re-orientation in the direction of permissiveness in order to cope with the problem of HIV/AIDS. Our position has also been one of total respect for confidentiality. But while maintaining confidentiality of the infected person, we have not hesitated to strongly advocate with him/her to refrain from violating the rights of others to remain uninfected as a result of his/her action. Whenever it has come to our knowledge, for instance, that an HIV positive person is about to marry an uninfected person without informed consent, we have prevailed upon the individual not to engage in what we see as an essentially exploitative act. While upholding the right of every person to marry, we also uphold the basic human right of every person not to be infected intentionally, or to be robbed of a healthy and long married life. Our awareness activities include urging individuals, parents and families to be cautious in this regard.

Overall, two perspectives govern our intervention in the area of HIV/AIDS. One is the gross gender injustice against women that HIV/AIDS highlights. We had to constantly sensitise and empower our team to address gender, whether in the rural setting, on highways, in sex work or in industry. It would have been easier to leave gender aspects alone, but we have consciously chosen to incorporate them as part of our health education programme on STDs and HIV/AIDS, as we found this to be a glaring gap in conventional approaches to HIV prevention. The other perspective relates to the strong link between poverty and vulnerability to HIV/AIDS. As incidence of HIV/AIDS grows among people below the poverty line, lost incomes and increased debt burdens accentuate pre-existing poverty. In this context, we find it difficult to talk about good nutrition and exercise and treatment of opportunistic infections, leave alone anti-retroviral treatment. Persons infected with HIV/AIDS lie terribly weakened or dying in the midst of already impoverished families. Working with these people over the years from early stages of their disease, and witnessing the hollow cheeks, empty stomachs and malnourished children among infected and uninfected alike, we stand helpless and unable to meet their economic needs. This is especially significant in those geographic regions where PREPARE does not already have a development programme. Every life is valuable and precious and has to be nurtured and saved. This has reinforced for us the importance of overall development – socio-political, gender, and economic – as the best medicine for HIV/AIDS.

SECTION THREE

Raising Awareness about Sexuality

An Overview

The word 'sex' is often used loosely to mean specific sexual acts or sexual behaviour in general. But in effect we tend to use the word 'sex' as a sort of holdall for the multiple aspects of what is actually *sexuality*. One of the spin-offs of the HIV/AIDS epidemic in India and the fact that HIV/AIDS is predominantly spread through the sexual route is that it has brought sexuality out of the closet for the first time in the country's recent history. And the word 'sexuality' itself is slowly coming into common parlance as a more appropriate usage for the whole gamut of sources of identity that makes us who we are as sexual beings. In this inclusive form, sexuality provides a framework within which to understand the feelings, thoughts, and actions that drive us.

At the base of sexuality is sex, which is the biological definition of a person's sexual identity as male or female. Sexuality also includes sexual behaviour, which comprises both specific sexual acts and the social contexts within which these acts take place. It encompasses subjective sexual identity and the accompanying bodily processes, emotions and passions, and types of sexual relationships with others that result from this identity. Finally, sexuality also includes gender, or the manner in which specific socio-cultural contexts shape what it is to be male or female, and the power equations between men and women. Sexuality, therefore, goes much beyond biology; it is shaped by society and culture, and in turn moulds motivations, perceptions and expectations, i.e., the way we perceive ourselves and behave as women and men. It involves choice, conflict and decision-making.

Seen thus, sexuality is all around us in subtle and not-so-subtle ways. In recent years, it has taken on a much more explicit character, particularly in the popular media. Print media stories have been turning the spotlight on sexuality from time to time. Depictions of sexuality in Indian films and music videos are becoming increasingly explicit. Globalisation of entertainment brings uncensored Western television channels into the home. Pornography has become much more easily available through video films and on the Internet. Recent reports of the use of cell phone cameras by adolescents to film and circulate explicit scenes of sexual acts, and of hidden video cameras to trap prominent persons in compromising sexual encounters make consumers of popular media increasingly familiar with public representations of sexuality. Advertising is another vehicle that uses sexuality-based images to sell products and in the process recast notions of sexuality in association with fashion which defines public notions of beauty, attractiveness and sex appeal projected, again, by the popular media. The pronounced sexual orientation being imparted to several traditional community-level dance festivals and to popular cinema music lyrics and the growing popularity of Valentine's Day celebrations in urban areas, are further testimonies of the market both creating and responding to the desire of Indians to give expression to their sexuality.

The fact, however, is that there is a mismatch between what the combined effect of HIV/AIDS and the sexual revolution calls for and young people's confidence in their own sexuality. In its most private and intimate manifestation at the level of the individual, sexuality in Indian society still remains a shadowy arena, a confused, deeply secretive and even shameful and furtive aspect of people's being, something that they fight shy of publicly speaking and learning about for fear of being judged in negative ways – sounding 'immoral' or not quite in keeping with 'Indian culture and tradition' or too 'modern' or 'Western' –, or being slighted or rejected. Although in the last few years a small proportion of the society that is educated, lives in metropolitan cities and is exposed to globalising influences has been able to break out of this mould, it continues to hold true for the vast majority of the country's population.

This culture of taboo and silence at the level of the individual impacts on both boys and girls, women and men in serious and negative ways. One of its implications is an absence of safe, non-judgemental and confidential spaces in which people, especially young people, can open up and seek information and understanding about what is happening to their bodies and emotions, sort out their doubts and confusions and evolve a positive and confident sexuality for themselves. At the present time, it is only under conditions of total anonymity that people find the courage to ask questions or admit to having problems. If at all sexuality is openly talked about, the tendency is to refer to the actions of others rather than oneself, and to dwell on negative and/or violent, i.e., 'immoral' acts, such as men demanding sex from women in return for material favours, boys dealing out disfigurement or death to girls who refuse to succumb to demands for romance or sex, molestation, rape, dirty jokes or prurient stories. This only serves to strengthen the notion of sexuality as a taboo area. Rarely is sexuality upheld as an important and positive source of physical and mental well-being.

In India, sexuality education was unknown before the advent of the HIV/AIDS epidemic. In those more modern educational institutions that sought to prepare adolescents for life as adults, the focus was on biological maturation and procreation as part of the biology syllabus. Even this was seen as being more relevant to adolescent girls with a view to preparing them for their future role as mothers. The teaching style was didactic, stressing simple biology and avoiding direct reference to sexuality or other 'sensitive' aspects, and had no room for airing questions or doubts. None of this was genuine sexuality education, as it made no reference to issues of gender, choice, decision-making or conflict, issues that are vital to understanding personal growth and maturation, and that also lie at the heart of tackling HIV transmission. The issue of whether schools should be taking responsibility for sexuality education since parents feel inadequate about engaging their children in such sensitive discussions, continues to be debated on television talk shows from time to time, but there is still considerable ambivalence about its value. Schools themselves still prefer biology textbook-oriented 'sex education' taught by reluctant teachers, rather than change over to a more thoroughgoing sexuality education and life skills training by trained counsellors.

The sexual revolution that is now sweeping across the country in tandem with the fast maturing HIV/AIDS epidemic ought to act as a definitive spur to take on board sexuality education for the young. This would involve creating a friendly and confidential environment for young people to access accurate information about sex and sexuality, and openly discuss their doubts and confusions without fear of censure. Some of the earliest and successful experiments with sexuality education in the initial stages of the HIV epidemic in India were led by medical doctors doing HIV-related research. School authorities permitted the doctors to speak to students since they saw a medical professional as the right agent to deal with what they saw as strictly physiological matters. The students themselves tended to remain passive as long as their teachers or principal were in the room. It was only when the authority figures left and the doors were closed behind them that the floodgates of doubts, uncertainties, confusions and questions would burst open. Clearly, there was a huge demand for information and discussion. Girls' questions would be about menstruation and marriage, while adolescent boys wanted direct information about sex and penetration and masturbation. Whenever written anonymous questions were invited, the response tended to be even more overwhelming.

Several international Conventions on the Rights of the Child and the Rights of Adolescents and Youth that have come into existence in the wake of the HIV/AIDS epidemic stipulate that the young have the right to enjoy the highest standards of health, and to receive the necessary information and ideas that can help them realise such a right. Research data from various parts of the world, too, show that imparting sexuality-related information to the young delays the initiation of sexual activity by adolescents, empowers them to retain control over their own bodies even in the face of adverse peer pressure, and encourages condom use by those who are already sexually active. Yet the popular belief among both educational and health care 'gate-keepers' continues to be that giving the young sexuality-related information and education will increase sexual activity, and thereby pose dangers to 'public morality'. In the context of HIV/AIDS, this means enhancing the vulnerability of the young to the risks of infection.

One of the most important and tragic outcomes of this vulnerability is the growing infection of Indian young women within marriage. Lack of HIV/AIDS awareness in Indian society at large particularly among boys and men, the high value placed on early marriage particularly of daughters, the pressures on newly married women to get pregnant and the growing awareness about the importance of ante-natal care are leading to a situation where more and more young married women coming to health centres for pregnancy check-ups are testing HIV positive.

A whole area of social research into sexual behaviour among a range of population groups in the society has come into being, spurred by concerns about the rapid spread of HIV/AIDS across the country. The realisation that those at greatest risk of HIV infection are women who lack power for sexual negotiation with male partners whether as married women or as prostitutes, and young people who are going through the throes of discovering their own sexuality and who tend to engage in sexual experimentation without knowledge of self-protection, has led many of these studies to focus on these two groups. The studies show that given the taboos on open discussion of sexuality, on talking about sexual feelings, confusions and doubts, or seeking help in grappling with worrying personal issues such as sexual identity or real or imaginary feelings of sexual inadequacy, boys may begin to seek out sexual experiences early in life (as early as 16 years of age), often in response to ridicule and prodding by peers to 'perform' and demonstrate their masculinity. These experiences may range from consuming pornography, to sexual experimentation with sex workers or with older married women ('aunties'), or sex with other boys or girls of their acquaintance. Alcohol and other substance abuse may accompany such experiments. Notions of masculinity and sexual pleasure as involving aggressiveness and sexual dominance over women often result in forced or violent sexual encounters with reluctant partners. And since most sexual encounters are spontaneous, condoms are conspicuous by their absence. There is also a significant lack of knowledge about condoms, and of how to procure them. Inhibitions in this regard also play their role. The result is unsafe sex, leading in many cases to unwanted pregnancy and attempts at abortion, and sexually transmitted infections. The tendency of sexually active boys to have multiple partners drawn from the different pools of potential partners in their pre-marital sexual experiments, as mentioned earlier, multiplies routes for HIV transmission. The resounding finding from a range of recent biomedical and social science research studies that, in India, marriage poses the greatest risk of HIV infection for young women, shows the potential of young men with unrevealed pre-marital sexual histories to infect their wives and, through them, their unborn children.

The above-described expressions of sexuality are largely grounded in the gender inequalities in Indian society that influence the way boys and girls are brought up as sexual beings. Boys and men express their sexuality in ways that society and culture deem 'manly', and which take the form of 'eve teasing' and intimidating girls, seeking out sex when they feel the need for it, and often punishing those who refuse to respond to their demands or overtures. Boys may also turn on other boys who are younger or appear submissive, the latter characteristic equated with girls as the inferior or weaker gender, and force them into sexual encounters which may gradually become routine. Girls and women, on the other hand, are expected to be what society deems 'feminine', i.e., ignorant about sexuality, 'innocent' and submissive, including in sexual relations. This leaves them highly vulnerable in relation to men, i.e., unskilled to negotiate sexual relations in their own favour even within marital unions, and at times trapped in unwanted and coercive pre-marital sexual relations. Although notions of sexuality are not cast in stone and undergo change as do other areas of social behaviour, the fact that they play out their role at so many levels, ranging from the most intimate to the most public, and interrelate with other social influences, make them very complex social phenomena.

The chapter that follows is the story of a telephone help line called Talking About Reproductive and Sexual Health Issues (TARSHI) that was started in New Delhi by a young clinical psychologist in the early days of the HIV/AIDS epidemic. The objective of the help line was to provide a safe and anonymous 'space' where people could ask for information and guidance on sexuality-related issues and problems. The larger environment in which the help line was begun was one where the only interventions for control of HIV/AIDS were serosurveillance (anonymous testing of blood samples of 'high risk' groups such as prostitutes and their clients and truck drivers), public messages of prevention, and targeting of 'high risk groups', i.e., commercial sex workers, truck drivers, professional blood donors and intravenous drug users. The identification of HIV with 'high risk' groups implied that the rest of the population could sit back and enjoy a false sense of immunity. The emphasis of the public messages was on safe sex, without an understanding of the context in which safety was being prescribed as a regular practice. In a social environment where people have little opportunity to talk about sexual feelings and doubts, how were they going to interpret what was 'safe' in the context of HIV/AIDS? Questions put by callers to the help line – overwhelmingly male – revealed that they thought that if heterosexual sex was unsafe, anal sex must be a 'safe' alternative. In fact, the questions revealed that there was a lot of male-to-male anal sex going on anyway. This was not seen as 'homosexuality', in the Western sense of the term, but as a form of '*masti*' or 'enjoyment', or simply as a sexual release, especially when willing female partners were hard to come by. The reluctance of the public messages to openly address the sexual behaviour of men who have sex with men and the dangers of unprotected anal sex in the context of HIV transmission was indirectly fostering this misconception. Again, young boys who were having unprotected sex with older married women or 'aunties' believed that they were 'safe', since their partners were either sterilised or were using some form of contraception. 'Safety' was clearly being seen here only as safety from the complications of unwanted pregnancy. Public messages that sex with multiple partners was unsafe were misinterpreted as a need to avoid only group sex or sex with several partners in the course of a single night.

The huge response to the help line reveals the extent of demand for information on matters pertaining to sex and sexuality. It also reveals the extent of wrong knowledge and confusion among boys and men – the main callers to the help line, women being too inhibited to ask questions – regarding the most basic facts about male and female physiology. TARSHI counsellors use every call to the help line as an opportunity to impart information about HIV/AIDS and its prevention. But TARSHI focuses on sexual well-being, i.e., more than simply freedom from negative factors such as fear, illness or infection. It views sexual health also in terms of freedom to savour, enjoy and fully experience a positive sexuality through access to a range of choices, and sees its own role as one of expanding choice through expanding people's field of awareness.

A Telephone Help Line for Sexuality

The Case of TARSHI

RADHIKA CHANDIRAMANI

It is almost a decade since TARSHI (Talking About Reproductive and Sexual Health Issues) has been working at its mission – primarily through a telephone help line – of empowering people of all ages with knowledge that can help them free themselves from confusions, misconceptions, fears, violence and infection in relation to their sexuality. TARSHI believes that reproductive and sexual health decisions cannot be isolated from the issue of sexuality, which, in turn, is central to personal identity and self-esteem. TARSHI's basic premise is that the fundamental right to a life of dignity subsumes the right to sexual well-being, and to a self-affirming and enjoyable sexuality. As an organisation and as a strategy, TARSHI's mission is to help people along the road to expanding and exercising their sexual and reproductive choices. Its programme is accessible to everyone irrespective of gender, age, community or class identity and sexual preference. It recognises the existence of gender, class and age-based inequalities in society, and the social and cultural contexts that affect sexual and reproductive choice and behaviour. Hence, its programmes and activities are especially for women and young people who are relatively more disadvantaged in terms of expressing their sexuality.

TARSHI was founded in Delhi in 1996. My training as a clinical psychologist and subsequent work experience had sensitised me to the enormous lack of information among people about sexuality issues. In the era of HIV/AIDS and its predominantly sexual mode of transmission, this seemed an area calling for urgent intervention. A telephone help line to address concerns about sexuality seemed an effective mode of intervention, and for the first several years this remained TARSHI's core work. This has since expanded to include research and publications, interactive sessions in schools, newspaper advice columns in two national newspapers and the establishment of The Sexuality and Rights Institute (in collaboration with CREA, an NGO in Delhi) and the South and Southeast Asia Resource Centre on Sexuality. What follows is a description of the TARSHI telephone help line on sexual and reproductive health matters. It outlines the challenges of working on sexuality issues and emphasises the need to integrate sexuality information within HIV prevention efforts. It also looks at the special needs of women and young people in general.

Talking about sex

The telephone help line service is free, and the languages used are Hindi (the language predominantly spoken in the Delhi region) and English. Callers are encouraged to speak in whichever of these two languages they are comfortable with. The help line is accessible during working hours, three days a week from Monday through Wednesday, between 10 a.m. and 4 p.m.

The help line provides its callers with easily digestible information, counselling on problematic issues, and referrals so that they may follow up on sexual or reproductive health problems that require resolution. Specially trained counsellors answer queries about sexuality, encourage callers struggling to air their concerns to talk at their own pace, and willingly discuss and work through complicated or complex feelings or predicaments that callers might wish to share. Confidentiality is assured at all times. Towards this end, callers are given code numbers that also allow for anonymity. They are assured that they are free to call back as often as they wish and are encouraged to cite their code numbers to help the counsellor quickly establish the caller's identity and to move into a smooth and continuous flow of dialogue with them. All calls received on the help line are documented for analysis and greater in-depth understanding of the problems and concerns expressed by the callers. It is this understanding that has led to TARSHI's publications. It has been our experience that most calls to the help line originate from within Delhi, extending at the most to the surrounding areas of Ghaziabad, Faridabad and Meerut. A very small number of calls come from other states. About a third of the callers are repeat callers, i.e., those accessing the help line more than once.

Callers to the help line tend to begin with concerns that may appear to be unrelated to the problem uppermost in their minds. A typical call from a male caller, for instance, might begin by asking about masturbation. It might then go on to wondering whether nocturnal emission is harmful. The caller might then reveal that he has noticed that when he engages in sexual contact with another person, the nocturnal emission becomes infrequent. What might finally emerge is that he has no regular sexual partner and that all his sexual contacts are casual and unprotected. This is the point at which we are able to direct the conversation towards safer sex, contraception and the issue of HIV infection.

Free and frank discussion of sexual and reproductive health issues through a help line pre-supposes complete trust between the caller and the counsellor. Callers need that safe space where they feel they can voice their true thoughts and feelings without fear of being judged or threatened with negative consequences to their individual or social well-being. A trained counsellor capable of transmitting a non-judgemental choice of words and tone of voice is the mainstay of such a telephone help line; the slightest suspicion of being judged negatively by the counsellor at the other end of the line – an imperceptible change in tone of voice, sudden drawing in of breath, an awkwardly long silence – could cause a caller to withdraw instantly. A counsellor must also be a person of immense skill both in terms of knowledge of and effective communication about sexuality. Issues relating to STDs,

HIV/AIDS, and sexual preferences and behaviour have an even greater sensitivity because of the stigma attached to them. The same holds true for sexual abuse.

Being non-judgemental is not to be confused with being value-free; it is not a situation of "anything and everything is fine". Values have an important place in counselling and sexuality-related work. The values that guide TARSHI and the work of its counsellors are those of safeguarding individual autonomy, safety, pleasure and sexual and reproductive health. There have been occasions when we have needed to state these values categorically to callers on our help line. And it has implied refusal of the kind of help the caller was seeking. For example, there have been callers who have wanted to know whether there was a 'safe' way to sexually abuse someone, i.e., commit the abuse without serious implications. These have been occasions when we have tried to engage the person in discussion, with a view to find out why he felt unable to engage his desired partner in a consensual way, making it very clear that sex without consent is abuse, and that we would not provide information that would help the caller to abuse someone.

Another key element in sustaining client confidence in the help line is anonymity, i.e., not inquiring about the caller's identity. This adds to people's sense of safety. Not many with problems are willing to admit, even to themselves, that they are in need of mental health counselling or, as in this case, sexual health services/counselling. Their willingness to admit this to others, i.e., publicly, does not even arise. This is one of the reasons that psychotherapists try to ensure that their consecutive clients do not meet each other on their way in and out of therapy sessions. An obvious advantage of a telephone help line like TARSHI is that it is easy for the client to retain anonymity. A telephone help line does not need to have caller identification in terms of name and addresses, i.e., particulars that locate or relate a person to a given space are irrelevant to the helping process. Moreover, the absence of face-to-face interaction further renders a client unidentifiable, either visually or in terms of social/class identity. These factors, perhaps, explain the popularity of the help line. If a client ever makes a repeat call, the counsellor has the means to refer back to the last conversation using the relevant code number. The code number is also useful for research and analysis of the information base generated through the help line.

To date, the TARSHI help line has answered more than 55,000 telephone calls. Of these approximately 80 per cent have been from men and 20 per cent from women. Only a small percentage – 10 per cent – relate to issues concerning HIV/AIDS infection, and these queries mostly pertain to the mode of spread. The most dominant clusters of questions are around sex, masturbation and the sexual organs. In keeping with TARSHI's policy of being proactive on such issues, counsellors use the opportunity afforded by having to answer elementary questions about sexual organs or the practice of masturbation to introduce the subject of safer sexual practices. They follow this up by raising the issue of HIV infection and its relationship with safer sex practices. This often leads to a discussion on whether and what the caller already knows about HIV/AIDS. In the process, counsellors seek to clarify many misconceptions on the part of the caller.

It is our finding that the myths and misconceptions originate from the prevailing social attitudes compounded, very often, by misinterpretation of public messages on the subject of HIV/AIDS. Our detailed analysis of a subset of 15,000 calls reveals a pattern that substantiates the above broad-brush description. More than 80 per cent of callers are men, ranging in age from 10-year-olds to 70-year-olds. The dominant motive of callers – 58 per cent of all calls – is to obtain elementary information about sexual organs and sexual activity, principally masturbation and sexual performance and conception and contraception. The second most important category of concerns – a little above one-third of all calls – pertains to orgasm, ejaculation, infertility, menstrual problems and infections. Only a tiny proportion – around 6 per cent – of all calls relate to problems of inter-personal relationships such as emotional and sexual compatibility.

We may conclude from the above that elementary knowledge about sex and the human anatomy – male as well as female – is absent among a large section of the population in the country. This holds for all age groups of both men and women. Given the lack of information at such a basic level, it is not surprising that issues concerning infection have barely entered their consciousness. Sexually transmitted diseases and reproductive tract infections were not at the top of the concerns voiced by the callers to our help line. This is not to say that these concerns are of no significance in the Indian context; simply, that they remain unexpressed at least through the medium of a telephone help line. It ought to be mentioned that there could also be the factor that the callers might want to first test the waters, i.e., the attitudes of the counsellors, before moving into what they perceive as very intimate revelations. The heavy load of callers to the help line, in fact, indicates pent-up demand. It highlights the need to bring the question of safe sex practices and sexual and reproductive health issues into the open, and make them an integral part of the discourse on sex and sexuality.

The absence of even elementary knowledge of basic bodily processes and sexual activity, coupled with the lack of public discourse on the subject, perpetuates wrong notions and risky practices. Misconceptions about masturbation and nocturnal emission, and fears of sexual inadequacies and imperfections have, at times, been the main reasons behind unprotected and risky sexual activity, as was borne out by many calls, especially from the male callers to the help line. The question of safety was regarded relevant only with respect to contraception and not infection. It is precisely because of this that those who practised anal sex (both in homosexual and heterosexual contexts) did not understand why protection from HIV and other infections was an issue. In fact some callers regarded anal sex as a method of contraception. Many such misconceptions also surround the issue of sexual activity during menstruation (preference for this as a means of contraception, without awareness of the accompanying heightened risk of HIV transmission) and the use of substances such as mustard oil and cosmetic lotions.

Communicating about sexuality is a challenging task in the Indian context where sex is a taboo subject. There is a general hesitation about discussing sex freely. Talking about it is considered to be uncouth, shameless and lacking in respectability. It is not surprising, therefore, that such an environment gives rise to a wide range of myths and prejudices. And any attempt at communicating messages about healthy and safe sex practices becomes a complex task and one that could result in unanticipated outcomes. Two examples illustrate the huge amount of thought, research and pre-testing among diverse audiences that is required before public messages relating to sexual activity are actually put into the public domain. A series of messages put out by the Government of India's National AIDS Control Organisation (NACO) in 1996 and 1997 and widely carried by the national newspapers advised people to "Stay away from multiple sex or use condoms". Many callers to the help line were sure that what 'multiple sex' meant was several partners in the space of one night. They believed that as long as they limited sexual activity to a single encounter a night they were safe, i.e., they did not need to use condoms. Quite clearly, the understanding that they were drawing from the message was that it was okay to change partners on different nights. This was exactly the opposite of what the NACO campaign intended to convey. Similarly, in 1997, the Tamil Nadu State AIDS Control Society put out a public interest advertisement depicting a harried looking and obviously married woman worrying, "He is late again. Is there someone else ...?" The advertisement then went on to enjoin men to "Always use a condom. That is the mark of a real man." This was interpreted by several consumers of the advertisement as advice to the 'real' man to enter into non-monogamous sexual relationships. Also, that condoms were relevant only when he had sex with 'other' women and not with his wife.

Besides their ambiguous words and imageries in the eyes of the public, another drawback of safe sex messages in India is that they have tended to focus almost exclusively on heterosexual encounters. The obvious interpretation that anyone would draw from this depiction – the more lurid among them being billboards with silhouettes of a man and a woman, with a skull-and-bones (symbol of danger) in the space between them – is that sexually transmitted diseases, reproductive tract infections, HIV/AIDS, etc., are contracted only through the heterosexual route. There were many instances of callers to the help line revealing that they did not consider sexual activity between men to be sexual acts. To them, the 'real' sexual act is only penile-vaginal intercourse. This has adverse consequences, particularly in the context of HIV/AIDS. The lack of public interest campaigns/advertisements regarding means of ensuring safer sex in same-sex sexual activity can only serve to perpetuate and strengthen the existing myths which ignore the need for safer sex practices. This is equally true of lesbians. Although the rates of female-to-female transmission of the HIV virus are believed to be considerably lower than in the case of male-to-male transmission, the threat of infection remains. The fact is that many lesbians in India continue to have sexual contact with men. Lesbians may also have partners who may be concurrently having sex with men; often they may be pushed into doing so due to the social premium placed on a heterosexual relationship, marriage and assertion of conjugal rights by men, and to the discrimination against lesbians in general. The threat of HIV/AIDS infection to lesbians, therefore, is equally real.

Young people and sexuality

The culture of silence about bodily processes, sex and sexuality weighs most heavily on young people in Indian society, leaving them particularly vulnerable to HIV infection. The hesitantly growing public opinion – at least in metropolitan towns – that sexuality education ought to be introduced into school curricula is not as simple as it sounds. It requires revolutionising teachers' outlooks and methods of engaging the young. We continue to live in a society where, even in metropolitan schools, simple biology lessons on the human anatomy are not taught properly because teachers find it embarrassing to discuss the reproductive system. TARSHI has received calls on its help line from students asking to be explained the features of the reproductive system over the telephone. The plea usually is, "Please explains this. The teacher did not explain it and I have to appear for a biology test tomorrow." In one instance, a group of students got together, switched on the speakerphone and read out from the prescribed biology text those portions that they wanted us to explain.

Many young people have phoned the TARSHI help line asking to know precise facts on menstruation. There have also been questions asking what exactly are sanitary napkins. One caller began by asking the counsellor the meaning of 'whisper'. When the counsellor answered that it was the act of speaking softly, the caller repeated her question. The counsellor tried to illustrate the meaning of the word 'whisper' by speaking very softly, explaining that this was what the word meant. The young caller did not give up. She patiently persisted, "No, no, you have not understood my question. I mean the whisper that is being advertised these days on the television". It was then that the counsellor understood that the caller was referring to a particular brand of sanitary napkins. Incredible as this may seem in the so-called modern day and age, it illustrates the huge burden of ignorance, confusion and uncertainty about their bodies that young people are forced to labour under in the absence of friendly and accurate sources of information. A leading newspaper from Delhi carried a report that many young people thought the condom was a pill used both by males and females to prevent pregnancy, another example of such ignorance.

A fifth of the callers to the help line are below 20 years of age, and a majority of them – close to 80 per cent – are boys. Even reproductive health programmes to the extent that they exist in the country – discussing issues such as contraception, reproductive tract infections and abortion – hardly cater to the needs of adolescents, focused as they are on the 'family planning needs' of married women. This omission is also due to the false assumption that adolescents do not have any real or immediate reproductive health needs. Social taboos on open discussion of sex mean that adolescent sexual needs are even less acknowledged. Calls to the TARSHI help line debunk all assumptions that adolescents are best left alone and 'uncontaminated' by explicit and accurate information about sex. Based on our experience of the questions that young people ask, their knowledge needs would appear to include a whole range of issues: information about bodily processes and functions, masturbation, nocturnal emission, erectile dysfunction, premature ejaculation, sexual acts and techniques, the relevance of foreplay, contraception, how to enhance sexual pleasure, homosexuality, HIV/AIDS infection, interpersonal relationships, emotional dependence and sexual abuse.

Almost two-thirds of adolescent callers begin their calls with queries about sexual organs and sexual performance. The males among them are most concerned about masturbation, and they have their own perceptions, explanations and fears about the effects of this practice. Loss in the bodily stock of semen is the most common cause of worry; similar fears tend to be voiced about nocturnal emission or, as they put it, "semen in urine". Boys demonstrate a huge interest in knowing more about women's bodies. Of particular interest is whether women, too, masturbate. Corresponding to their own concerns about the size of the penis in relation to the ability to perform sexually is their concern about the significance of female breast size in terms of women's sexual desire and sexual satisfaction. Girls, on the other hand, do not demonstrate much interest in male sexual organs or desires (possibly out of shyness, again). Their concerns centre on breast size, menstrual irregularities, conception and contraception. Both young women and men have expressed concerns about inter-personal relationships.

Women and HIV/AIDS

That the culture of silence sits more heavily on girls and women than on boys and men is further substantiated by the fact that women callers are few in comparison with men, and that even fewer among them ask questions about HIV/AIDS, their questions dominated by concerns regarding conception and contraception. We may conjecture that the apparently low levels of interest in HIV/AIDS are because women perceive themselves to be at a low risk of infection. The more likely explanation is that they have no clue about the way in which HIV/AIDS could affect their lives.

The culture of silence that keeps women ill-informed on matters of sexuality and their bodies makes them even more wary than men about seeking information, even when the opportunity presents itself in the form of a relatively protected environment such as an anonymous telephone line. Several women who used the TARSHI help line began by expressing their reservations to the counsellor about the decorum of what they were doing, i.e., talking to strangers about intimate matters. They would begin by saying that it was only after much hesitation that they were accessing the help line; that they were not sure if it was proper for a woman to verbalise matters relating to sex; that it was important for them to know whether they were the only ones, i.e., whether the help line was at all accessed by other women. Many women callers – presumably married – told the counsellor that they were on the help line only at the prompting of their husbands; that their husbands had in turn assured them that the help line was a 'safe' one, i.e., staffed by female counsellors, with the promise of complete confidentiality and anonymity. Several of these women were responding to the advertisement of the TARSHI help line as being particularly responsive to women's concerns. Some even told the counsellor that their husbands had checked out the help line, rather like carrying out a pre-test of the service.

After initial hesitation is overcome and a certain level of comfort is reached about continuing the dialogue, women do start talking about those aspects of sexual behaviour that make them vulnerable to HIV/AIDS infection. What begins to emerge clearly is the difficulties women face in practising safer sex: that it is the male partner who dictates their sexual lives; that women rarely have a say in determining even the frequency of sex; and that their male partners refuse to take no for an answer. Many women callers complain of the resentment and harassment – physical violence and/or emotional harassment through taunts and other forms of abusive behaviour – by their male partners when they do not immediately respond to the demand for sex.

Women also express helplessness in getting men to use condoms. The usual response from men is either to accuse the women of being unfaithful, or to refuse on the grounds that condoms come in the way of sexual pleasure. The counsellors at TARSHI have at times posed the question to a number of male callers: do condoms compromise on sexual pleasure and if so how? Invariably, the answer they receive is that the men themselves have never used a condom, but have heard from friends that condoms come in the way of sexual pleasure.

An interesting form of sexual behaviour that has surfaced on the help line is what might be termed the 'aunty syndrome'. This is the phenomenon where young unmarried men, most of them in their late teens and early twenties, enter into sexual relationships with married, older women in the neighbourhood, women whom these young men usually address as 'aunty'. Aunties are usually in their mid or late thirties. An aunty enters into a sexual liaison with a young boy who is socially accessible to her. Sex takes place when the woman's husband is away at work or is travelling. These aunties continue to have sex with their husbands who, in turn, may or may not be monogamous. Judging by the accounts of callers to the help line, aunties would seem to be using some form of contraception, usually the oral contraception pill, intra-uterine device or tubectomy.

Talking to young men beset by the 'aunty syndrome', we have found ourselves having to address many issues at different levels, issues of power, safety, guilt, moral considerations and sexual codes. Interwoven through all these are the callers' assumptions about the woman and her husband – as decent, clean, nice and respectable people, overall presenting a picture of a 'good family' that cannot be affected by HIV. It takes a number of calls before the issue of HIV/AIDS can be seriously taken up for discussion. The young men caught in the 'aunty syndrome' begin to make calls to the help line when they want to opt out of their liaisons, either because they are about to get married, or because the aunty has become excessively demanding of attention and time or because the liaison is threatening to become socially risky or because the boys are just fed up with the relationship. Aunties react strongly to any suggestion of a break-up, ranging from reprimands to issuing threats of social exposure on grounds of attempted molestation. As far as the counsellors on the help line are concerned, all the stories are one-sided, and there is no way of checking out the aunties' side of the stories. No aunty has hitherto ever called the help line to seek counselling in the matter. These sexual liaisons have significance with respect to HIV/AIDS infection. The aunties do not see the need for condom use because they practice other forms of contraception. The boys listen to the aunties because they regard them as knowledgeable on matters of sex. Aunties continue to have sex with their respective husbands alongside the liaisons, and it is possible that the husbands in turn have other sexual contacts. These are precisely the kinds of issues that the TARSHI help line brings to the notice of those not so well informed.

Working against the odds

Working on sexuality issues is a complex, challenging and often frustrating task. It is also deeply personal, in the sense that it raises many questions that have ethical and social implications for one's work. To give an example of just some of the dilemmas we face: do we as counsellors withhold or share information on calls originating from cranks? Whose rights and privileges do we trade-off? Above all, we work in the field of sexuality within a cultural context that is sexually repressive, a culture that equates sex with a notion of shame, where decorum (*sharam*) for women is defined as submission, and holding back from seeking help. Because we provide information and help on matters pertaining to sexuality, some judge us as *besharam*, women who are themselves lacking in decorum. There was a time when we were inundated with calls from men who thought that ours was a sex line, along the lines of party and chat lines. We even had to resort to installing an answering machine to announce that TARSHI was not a sex or 'friendship' line. Now only a small percentage of our calls – less than 10 per cent – are from pranksters. But when a spate of such episodes occurs, they could prove upsetting for the help line staff.

Ours is also a service where the burnout syndrome sets in early and often with magnified effect. Burnout symptoms surface when counsellors become noticeably mechanical in their work, start showing apathy towards callers' problems or become cynical about the possibility of callers resolving the problems for which they access the help line. Some counsellors become increasingly incapable of facing up to the deeply personal reverberations triggered off by the very nature of our work. Some start showing a distinct lack of willingness to learn and adapt to the new challenges thrown up in the course of their work.

One of the reasons is the nature of the work, which is both demanding and stressful. Adding to the stress and fatigue of the job is the fact that we have no way of receiving feedback from our callers, no way of knowing whether we have been successful in answering their need for help, or whether the information that we imparted was at all imbibed. A sizeable proportion of our callers convey feelings of frustration, despair, intention to abuse, or fear of the threat of abuse. We try through the help line to help them regain their balance. We work through with them possible courses of action that they can take on their own, and we provide names and addresses of agencies and institutions that can provide greater help if required, whether legal or social. However, we rarely get to know whether the desperate or anguish-ridden situation was resolved at all. The principles of anonymity and confidentiality under which we operate put restrictions on how far we can go, which becomes a cause of emotional and mental stress to the counsellors, adding to their concerns about callers' well-being. Counsellors are privy to reports of incest, domestic violence and other forms of sexual and mental abuse. As counsellors, they are required to respond professionally, without becoming emotionally involved. This is not easy for every counsellor to come to terms with, and often a certain sense of helplessness and frustration sets in.

Conceptual clarity, maintaining an emotional distance from those who seek our service and striking the right balance between patience and compassion are all essential requirements for counselling work of this nature. That these are difficult traits to impart, acquire and sustain is evident from the high attrition rate among our counsellors. This is a source of considerable worry for TARSHI. Identifying suitable candidates, training and retaining them remains one of the on-going challenges to the sustainability of the help line. Counsellors are trained to identify and deal with symptoms of burnout and undergo periodic refresher trainings as a way of sustaining morale. We need also to be able to innovate a much wider range of mechanisms that can overcome the problem of premature burnout that currently afflicts sexual counselling work.

Fundamental to the work at TARSHI is the value we place on our counsellors' sense of self-esteem, both as persons and as professionals. We have come up with some rough and ready ways of keeping the negative aspects of the work at bay. These include regular discussions within the group that cover the issues faced individually and collectively by the members of the team. The discussions may range from a dissection of a particularly knotty problem as presented by a caller, to a discussion of whether new factual knowledge is required, to reviewing a standard way of approaching an issue with a view to coming up with better or alternative ways of responding to the expressed needs of callers. These meetings are also important platforms for sharing the sorts of feelings that many calls tend to trigger off. We also chip in for each other when there is need for one of us to overcome an episode of discomfort or depression or a sense of failure. We have a system of ongoing training and supervision. We make group presentations and have book review sessions. We also make attempts to create a feeling of fellowship by celebrating birthdays and anniversaries within the group, holding parties and going on retreats, all meant to relieve the tedium of responding to calls on the help line.

One of the great difficulties we face is when the need arises to make a referral. There are occasions when we know that a caller needs professional help from someone in the legal or medical community, but it is a big challenge to identify expert advice and help from professionals who are sensitive about sexuality issues. So far we have not come across any network in this regard. What acts as an obstacle is the widely prevalent negative attitude towards the problems of those who are either poor, or who belong to a sexual minority group, or who are HIV positive.

There is, however, a discernible wind of change for the better. A decade ago when TARSHI first started its work it was a lonely existence for us. There was an element of tentativeness, a defensive stance to our existence. In fact, we felt compelled to take cover by describing our work in the most general terms, i.e., concern for young people's health, violence against women and reproductive health issues. Sexuality was like a sub-text. Today, the scene has changed. The push for this change has come from NGOs, social activists – mostly women – and, to a lesser extent, from the media. Today, much more information on sexuality is available openly, particularly in the media. It may not always be the most accurate information on the subject, but that it has come to occupy some space in the public discourse is a significant development. HIV/AIDS prevention efforts inevitably bring sexual practices into open discussion. Also, in the last five years or so, there has been a mushrooming of many more help lines on HIV/AIDS, violence and lesbian and gay issues. TARSHI currently hosts the secretariat of a national network of help lines and is no longer a lone voice in the wilderness.

SECTION FOUR

HIV/AIDS and Women in Prostitution

An Overview

Since the onset of the HIV/AIDS epidemic in the country, women in sex work have borne the worst brunt of the unchecked spread of the virus. Their burden has been both physiological and social. Physiologically, as a group, they suffer the highest levels of HIV infection in the country due to their extreme vulnerability to the virus. Socially, their stigmatisation as 'fallen women' has worsened in the context of HIV due to the spotlight being turned on them as the 'principal vectors' – or main carriers – of the infection. Both burdens raise major questions of social and economic justice and gender rights, for at the core of the condition of women in prostitution are issues of gender, sexual and economic inequalities. Therefore, no discussion of them as 'target groups' in relation to HIV can take place outside of this context.

The markers of vulnerability to HIV transmission are: a high rate of partner change, pre-existing untreated sexually transmitted infections, and unprotected sexual intercourse. In India, women in prostitution are prey to all three markers. The bulk of these women are in prostitution because they are poor, uneducated, and unskilled. They are often married, but are unsupported by alcoholic husbands or forced into prostitution by violent husbands or have simply been deserted. Therefore, in order to eke out a living, they need to take on several low-paying clients.

Poverty also keeps them in a state of poor health and nutrition, and with little access to prompt, effective and non-discriminatory treatment for repeated sexually transmitted infections. Finally, it is only when clients use condoms that women in prostitution can protect themselves from contracting HIV. But in order to negotiate condoms with male clients whose main demand is 'skin-on-skin' sex, women in prostitution need to know about HIV/AIDS and the importance of condoms, they need to develop negotiation skills, and they need to be organised as a group to insist on condom use so that their individual livelihoods are not jeopardised.

Depending on the nature of their economic servitude, women in prostitution may work in brothels in bondage to *gharwalis* (brothel keepers), or as semi-independent sex workers under the control of pimps, or as self-employed women/housewives. Regardless of the nature of their work organisation, their stigmatised social status leaves them constantly open to exploitation by police and local criminals (*goondas*) at whose hands they suffer physical violence, monetary extortion and coercion into unsafe sex as the price for 'protection' from the imprisonment. Abetting these violent assaults is an ambiguous legal framework that criminalises women in prostitution.

The law does not make prostitution *per se* or the visiting of prostitutes by men illegal, but deems running of a brothel, practising prostitution in the vicinity of a "public place", soliciting or "seducing" in a "public place" or living off the earnings from prostitution to be illegal. The Immoral Traffic (Prevention) Act of 1956 that was brought into existence ostensibly to prevent the exploitation for commercial gain (trafficking) of women and children (girls under 16 years) by pimps and brothel keepers, gives the police and the courts wide-ranging powers. It gives them the discretion to decide if a person is a prostitute and then remove her from "any" place and prohibit her from re-entering it on pain of imprisonment. The police may search any premises they suspect of being used for prostitution and arrest women whom they identify as 'prostitutes' without any search or arrest warrants; a woman who resists such a search of her premises is deemed to have committed a cognizable offence and may be arrested. The police may hold arrested women in custody until they are able to produce them before the "appropriate" magistrate. Magistrates are empowered to pass orders in keeping with the Indian Penal Code for the imprisonment of women they deem 'prostitutes' for any period between two and five years.

The Act thus gives power to the 'guardians of law and order' to arbitrarily render women in prostitution invisible as dangers to 'decent' society. This they do by segregating them into ghettos ('red light areas'), even while their clients proliferate among the 'guardians' of 'public morality'. It is also common for the police to resort to verbal threats and humiliation of women in prostitution, and periodically book them as criminals on petty charges such as trespassing (into a 'public place') or 'indecent exposure', or on trumped up charges of being in possession of narcotics, or for the purpose of 'rescuing' them from brothels for 'rehabilitation' or for being in possession of condoms which is used as a handle to accuse the women of soliciting for sex. All these encounters with the law enforcement agencies are accompanied by pressures on the arrested women to admit to charges, followed by the imposition of fines and bribes in lieu of being jailed, thus adding to the circle of corruption. These encounters are not only economically taxing for the women concerned (forcing them to entertain even more clients to make up the losses); they are also full of possibilities for violence against the women and, especially, sexual abuse. The implications of the criminalisation of sex work for HIV transmission is that it leaves women in prostitution even more vulnerable to the infection and reduces their bargaining power to consistently negotiate condoms with every partner. The Immoral Traffic (Prevention) Act was revised in 1987 with a view to add more stringent clauses for the protection of children and minors. Yet, it has not made a dent on the Indian child-sex industry, which is believed to be one of the largest in the world.

Women in sex work were identified early in the Indian epidemic as a high risk group. However, while promiscuous male clients were seen as needing protection from the virus, the women came to be targeted as the source of infection; indeed, society itself was seen as needing protection from them. The first official responses to the identification of the HIV virus were the Tamil Nadu government's imprisonment of infected sex workers, and the Maharashtra government's deportation of south Indian women in sex work back to Tamil Nadu and Karnataka.

It is only with the passage of time, and largely as a result of pressure from Indian NGOs and international donor agencies supporting the Government of India's HIV/AIDS intervention projects, that women in prostitution and sex work have come to be recognised as also deserving of protection, and are now included in condom campaigns. They are now exhorted by the National AIDS Control Organisation to assist in HIV/AIDS control through enforcing universal condom use among their peers. Several groups of such women across the country have eagerly responded to the call. For the first time, they see themselves as being accorded citizenship status as partners in a national cause. They also find it encouraging to see that government has begun to recognise the crucial importance of mutual responsibility of sexual partners, whether inside or outside of marital unions.

However, NACO's hand of partnership is yet to make an impact upon society's stigmatisation of sex workers, or harassment and sexual exploitation by the police. Women in sex work still find the doors of mainstream hospitals and doctors routinely closed to them. The latest excuse for police threats and arrests of women in prostitution has become the possession of a condom. And organised condom promotion work by sex workers under the umbrella of the National AIDS Control Programme is now beginning to be seen by powerful local elites – always males – as an attempt by these marginalised and criminalised women to claim social legitimacy and, therefore, pose a threat to the social and moral order of which the men see themselves as the self-appointed guardians.

Understanding the gender, sexual and economic exploitation suffered by women in prostitution offers a window to the social veil of double standards that subjugate women's sexuality in general – whether they are in prostitution or in households – to the demands of men. The double standards grant men sexual licence before and after marriage on grounds that it is in keeping with their biological nature. On the other hand, the double standards reward as 'virtuous' women who unquestioningly submit their sexuality to the demands of men within marriage. Even married women who seek to exercise control over their own sexuality, i.e., are unwilling to give in at all times to husbands' demands, face the danger of being branded 'immoral' and being forced to submit. Women in prostitution who are in relatively greater charge of their own sexuality outside of the institution of marriage are only the other side of the same coin of gender inequality. These double standards have huge implications for women's ability in general to negotiate sexual relations with dignity and safety.

The significance of SANGRAM's inclusion in this collection of essays is that it illustrates many of these complexities. SANGRAM, an NGO based in Sangli district in the interior of Maharashtra state, started off as the courageous choice of one middle class professional woman to focus on organising women in prostitution in the context of HIV/AIDS as active agents of their own health and human rights. The initiative led to the establishment of a collective of women in prostitution and sex work – Veshya AIDS Mukabla Parishad or VAMP – administered and run by the women themselves with guidance from the parent organisation. Today, the work of the two partner NGOs that covers awareness-raising about HIV/AIDS, sexuality and gender relations, has extended beyond women in sex work within cities and districts in southern Maharashtra and northern Karnataka to include married household women in rural areas (who are vulnerable to HIV due to their husbands' possibly irresponsible behaviour), and among young adults and adolescent boys and girls in the region, both in and out of school and college. This extension of coverage is significant. Research in many parts of the country among less educated and economically disadvantaged communities shows that marriage has become the single most important risk factor for young women.

Despite SANGRAM/VAMP's low profile and sustained and commendable work – today, virtually no woman engaged in sex work in that region will entertain a client who refuses to use a condom –, they have had their share of persecution by local police and elites. Most recently in February 2002, the VAMP collective purchased a house and the property on which it was situated in Nippani, a small town in Karnataka. This was planned as the organisation's base for conducting meetings and planning and executing their HIV/AIDS prevention work. Very soon, objections to their visibility were being raised by local political influentials, who used verbal threats followed by violence on their property and person in order to evict them from the area. When VAMP leaders attempted to file a police report complaining against the violence, the police refused to admit the report. Colluding with the politicians and the town's elected officials, the police contended that as prostitutes the women had no civil rights as they were not "normal citizens", implying thereby that they did not have the right to personal freedom or security, or freedom from physical or sexual abuse. The men accused the women – including the founder of SANGRAM – of using HIV to run a brothel, and adduced condom distribution as evidence of this. They threatened to "strip (the women) in the public square and beat (them) black and blue" and charge them under the "immoral traffic" law. VAMP's office and the homes of its leaders were vandalised, the women were dishoused, and their condom distribution work was stopped. The incident acquired national and international media visibility. Protest rallies were held, both in Sangli (the headquarters of SANGRAM) and in Nippani by women's groups and human rights groups, and the government was pressured to appoint an official enquiry into the matter. What the incident did highlight, forcefully, was the bind in which hitherto invisibilised and marginalised groups now find themselves in relation to both their own citizenship rights and their HIV/AIDS prevention roles.

Admittedly, most women in prostitution are not in it as a result of choice. However, once they are within the trade, neither their civil nor socio-economic rights and nor indeed any larger social purpose is served if they are simply perceived as vile, outcast or criminal and, therefore, further marginalised. What they need – like other citizens in the polity – is to be empowered to exercise control over their own bodies and life circumstances. HIV/AIDS has helped raise this issue of citizenship and responsibility for the first time, particularly in relation to marginalised groups. HIV intervention work has brought into existence several sex worker collectives/organisations. A major demand of these groups is for the decriminalisation of prostitution. This is a demand first and foremost for change of the laws relating to prostitution, so that women who have to earn their livelihood through sex may do so in safety, and without stigmatisation. This means, above all, freedom from arbitrary violence and sexual exploitation at the hands of the police in the name of protecting law and order and protecting 'virtuous' women and children from 'wanton women'. It also means freedom from manipulation and slavery at the hands of criminal syndicates that seek to traffic in women and children in order to reap profits out of the sale of female bodies. The multimillion-dollar international criminal rackets that sell women and children into prostitution across national borders ultimately feed off society's unreformed gender and economic disadvantages that deny women rights over their own bodies.

Groups across the world that are working for the human rights of women in sex work argue that the citizenship rights of women in prostitution are as important as the rights of any other section of civil society that follows its own trade or business. They argue for a worldview that places personal responsibility at the centre of its scheme of values; that taking responsibility for one's sexual actions is one component of taking responsibility for oneself and all of one's actions, something that applies to all citizens. The HIV epidemic has helped focus not just on individual responsibility, but also on mutual and collective responsibility in the interests of the social good. It is this principle that women in sex work are articulating when they refuse to entertain a customer without the mutual protection of a condom, thus elevating the HIV/AIDS prevention programme from a mere condom distribution exercise to a discourse on civil and human rights for all.

Organising Women in Prostitution

The Case of SANGRAM

MEENA SESHU

SANGRAM, based in Sangli in the state of Maharashtra, was one of the earliest NGOs to step into the field of HIV/AIDS prevention, focusing exclusively on women in prostitution and sex work. SANGRAM was initially drawn to this constituency because women in prostitution and sex work had emerged as a critical group in relation to HIV/AIDS, demonstrating alarmingly high rates of infection. Women in prostitution and sex work were also being identified in the scientific literature as a 'high risk group' in the context of HIV transmission, and their clients as a 'bridge population' in relation to the general heterosexual population, i.e., an important intermediary group where men who contracted the infection passed it on to their wives or other female partners. The government's approach towards this already socially marginalised and stigmatised community was to simply label women in prostitution and sex work as 'vectors' of the disease, and stigmatise and criminalise them further on this account. From its earliest response of imprisoning women in prostitution and sex work in order to 'protect' society from them, official policy gradually evolved to one of listing them among the high-risk groups, and targeting them for condom use.

SANGRAM's approach to the issue of women in prostitution and sex work in relation to HIV transmission was, from the start, a self-consciously different one from the above. It saw them as being as much in need of protection as the rest of mainstream society. If their lives and health were valuable in their own right, the task then was to find out how they might be empowered to protect themselves in their own interests, and thereby contribute to the social good. This implied mainstreaming issues of women in prostitution and sex work, something that had never been attempted before.

Over the years, this approach has evolved into the establishment of an independent collective of women in prostitution that now engages in HIV/AIDS prevention work as a partner of the government in the National AIDS Control Programme. In this partnership, women in prostitution and sex work see themselves as playing a valuable social role in a national cause. SANGRAM's fostering role in the emergence and stabilisation of the collective goes beyond a strategic focus within the context of the HIV/AIDS epidemic. It forcefully articulates a conceptual framework relating to women in prostitution that extends to larger issues of gender, sexuality and society. This framework is intended to guide its efforts over the long term to bring issues of sex workers in from outside the pale.

In the interim, the struggle to simply sustain the presence of women in prostitution and sex work within the government's HIV/AIDS programme is an ongoing one, given the huge and deeply ingrained stumbling block of societal rejection. Paradoxically, even as women in prostitution and sex work are becoming part of the government's prevention campaign, their stigmatisation takes on ever more complex forms. Their poverty, sex worker status and gender had always gone against them. Targeting them as vectors in HIV transmission only added to the burden of stigma. Now, their role in promoting condom use as part of their AIDS prevention work is used against them by the police to arbitrarily harass or arrest them on grounds of soliciting, thus criminalising them.

Early beginnings of the organisation

The 'devadasi districts'

SANGRAM began its work in 1992 in Sangli district in Maharashtra, one of the districts in the country identified as the worst hit by the HIV virus. The organisation has over the years extended its reach to four adjacent districts in the state – Satara, Kolhapur, Solapur, and parts of Pune in Maharashtra – as well two districts in the neighbouring state of Karnataka.

SANGRAM's constituency consists of women who belong to communities clustered in the border region of Maharashtra and Karnataka that have traditionally followed sex work as an income-earning activity. Sex work in this region is an offshoot of the traditional *devadasi* system that has historically been a cultural feature of these inter-state border districts. The institution continues to endure there, with a visible presence of women who are routinely dedicated to the profession by their natal families. Whole villages share the *devadasi* sub-culture, and are interconnected by social networks that initiate and sustain new entrants into the business, and take care of those who retire from it.

The most distinctive characteristic of the *devadasi* system is that it represents a symbiosis between the coping strategies of families in extreme poverty, temple patronage that traditionally fed off the vulnerability of the women among the poor, and the fact that these women also became very powerful due to their sexual proximity to the leaders in the village. An extremely poor household could offer a daughter in the service of the goddess – consecrate her as a *devadasi*, a 'handmaiden of the goddess' –, and the temple management thereafter took over the responsibility of meeting her material needs from the revenues accruing to the temple. The girls so offered danced before the gods, and became prey to sexual exploitation by those who were influential in the temple management or village social structure. Over time, the system became further vitiated into one of rampant exploitation, leading to the institutionalisation of the system in the form of prostitution. The system thrived because of older *devadasis* who used the system to gain money, power and status in the village.

No contingent of *devadasis* exists as part of temple systems any more. However, the religious panoply of the practice continues in a new variant. Families in extreme poverty now tie a pendant of particular design around the neck of daughters to symbolise their status of being left entirely on their own to fend for themselves. These women then seek security with other women from their own kin group, village, or circle of friends who preceded them similarly into the sex trade. This readymade group of peers with kin or village ties provides some cushion against the severe trauma of being initiated into sex work. Another distinctive characteristic of this group is that they do not lose their families by virtue of their work. Rather, they continue to maintain close and regular links with parents, siblings and extended family networks, visiting them often, carrying gifts for them, and generally being economically valuable members of their families by regularly remitting money. Most of the women with whom SANGRAM works fall within this category.

SANGRAM first came into existence in the early 1990s when the HIV/AIDS scare was just gathering momentum. In 1986 when HIV/AIDS was first reported in Maharashtra, the state government had set up a committee which suggested that 'high risk groups' such as women in prostitution and sex work and transport workers should be targets for intervention. Of the total HIV/AIDS cases in Maharashtra, 97.5 per cent were a result of unprotected heterosexual sex. Condom distribution and raising awareness about protected sex through condom use among the above-mentioned high-risk groups (also described as core-transmitters of the virus), was considered to be the most potent weapon against the spread of HIV/AIDS. Government-sponsored district-level Societies were formed to concentrate on high prevalence areas like Mumbai, Pune, Sangli and Kolhapur – all major towns in the state.

Sangli's special prominence in terms of HIV incidence is due to several factors. Among the more important is its geographical location close to the Maharashtra-Karnataka border.

The two towns of Sangli and Miraj form a central junction for southern Maharashtra and northern Karnataka. Located on the rim of the vast rural hinterland that extends into both states, they are both easily accessible by both road and rail. The Sangli-Miraj corridor has a high concentration of hospitals and clinics, which attract patients from the neighbouring towns and cities. Routine HIV testing by all doctors has become the norm for any minor ailment, especially for surgery, irrespective of whether there is a need for the HIV test. Part of the reason for Sangli showing up high figures of HIV infection could well be this factor. Sangli town has the added feature of being one of the major urban centres for *devadasi* migration, and women in prostitution and sex work have a high visibility in the town. Sangli thus represents the urban-rural-rural spread of the epidemic in the state.

The birth of SANGRAM

I had moved to Sangli from Mumbai in the early 1990s soon after taking my Master's degree in social work, as my first step towards fashioning a career as a social activist. Initially, I worked as a journalist as I found journalism effective for focusing public attention on social issues. In the course of my work I became intrigued by what appeared to be the unique position of Sangli in the context of the emerging HIV epidemic. The early negative focus on women in prostitution and sex work as 'vectors' of HIV, the clear vulnerability of these women to HIV/AIDS, and the positive feature of their cultural cohesiveness, all prompted me to begin thinking in terms of how I might work with them, thereby putting my training in social work to good effect. I was greatly helped by Dr. Vijay Thakur whose conceptual clarity on issues of women in prostitution helped fashion the collectivisation model adopted by SANGRAM.

I surmised that without a formal organisational set-up and legal standing for garnering financial support, I would have little basis for an enduring engagement with these women. Casting around for what might be the most appropriate point of entry, I learnt of a dormant NGO in Sangli that was already registered with the Government of Maharashtra as a 'Society' of individual members, and as a Public Trust. The NGO's general objective of working with disadvantaged women coincided with my own. I requested for a meeting with its Board members to explain my proposed mission. They enthusiastically welcomed the initiative as they felt that the inactive organisation would now serve its stated objective well. With neither any deadweight to clear, nor any imposition of conditions for the take-over, I was saved the time and effort involved in registering a new organisation, and was able to start work immediately. My first steps were to recast the specific objectives of the organisation to suit the particular needs of the women in prostitution whom I had identified as my primary constituency, and to bring together a new group of Trustees who were sympathetic to my concerns and willing to participate actively in the management of the organisation. I chose to use the acronym – SANGRAM – of the original registered name (Sampada Grameen Mahila Sanstha translated as Village Women's Organisation).

SANGRAM signifies 'The Battle'. And battle it was indeed from the very start. My first opponents were the very people whom I wanted to befriend, the sex workers themselves. As hardnosed a group as one might find anywhere, mistrust was their watchword. These women had encountered so many fly-by-night-do-gooders that they had lost all faith in both individuals and civil society at large.

I had to begin my work entirely alone. My expectation as a young social work graduate had been that as a woman other women, particularly those who were considered by many as society's rejects, would greet me with open arms. I had expected them to be wildly enthusiastic about my self-professed mission as a social worker to organise them into a collective, and had fantasies of them flocking to the discussions and group meetings I was attempting to organise. On the contrary, they cold-shouldered me. I was in their midst everyday, longing to be accepted as a well-wisher, but found that I was an irritant and avoidable intrusion instead. In fact, my daily presence seemed actually to be disturbing them and their clients. But I persisted, seizing every opportunity to explain why I was there. The inevitable question that they threw at me each day was, "What is so special about you that we should trust you?" I found to my discomfiture that this was a question to which I had no foolproof answer.

I was trying, additionally, to cope with my own frustration at having to tolerate the foul-mouthed behaviour of the men who lounged around in the labyrinthine lanes of the 'red light' areas. These men were simply unable to stomach the presence of a middle-class woman in their area. One day one of them came up to me and roughly demanded sex, as if it was the only logical explanation for my daily presence there. I was in tears, my morale virtually shattered. And I was indignant. Nothing that I had learnt in my social work training had prepared me for this.

The episode, however, proved to be the catalytic agent for the cooperative relationship I had been seeking to establish between these women and myself. The women responded to the men's slighting of me with spontaneity and generosity. They now became my protectors and patrons. Aprava *mausi,* an aunt-like authority figure in the area, said to me indulgently and comfortingly, "Forget it. Think of the meeting that I am organising for you tomorrow." She waited for me to smile at her through my tears. My work had begun. Aprava *mausi* was to become the fulcrum of our activities and the role model for several who chose to follow in her footsteps. They became SANGRAM.

Building up SANGRAM

Building capacity through a cadre of peer educators

Aprava *mausi* ran a brothel in Gokul Nagar, one of the colonies of women in prostitution and sex work in Sangli. Aprava *mausi* is a *gharwali. Gharwalis* are women who were once in prostitution themselves, but who are now retired due to advancing age. As opportunities for sex work began to diminish, they had the sagacity to invest in a house or two, and provide shelter and other forms of support to younger women for a fee. The fee, which is called 'commission', is fixed at 50 per cent of the earnings of the girl. Some *gharwalis* have their own sisters and daughters living with them and doing sex work. For me, *gharwalis* became the obvious point of reference, the recruiters or recommenders for the pool of peer educators I was trying to put together. They themselves could not be the peer educators, as the criterion that I had fixed for a peer educator was that she should be an active sex worker herself.

As mentioned earlier, the starting point of SANGRAM's work among women in prostitution and sex work was the threat of the HIV/AIDS epidemic, with a strong emphasis on condom distribution and use. However, SANGRAM's philosophy that gradually came to be shared among the growing group of local adherents did not subscribe to the view that women in prostitution and sex work were the most potent carriers of HIV/AIDS. It was true that the impact of the epidemic could take its most severe form among sex workers; they could suffer high levels of infection and re-infection, bear HIV/AIDS infected children and languish in total hopelessness for want of counselling and care. However, it was also our understanding, strengthened by a growing exchange of views with NGOs in India and other parts of the world, that women in prostitution can be very reliable enforcers of condom usage, and that they are also good educators for their clients. We could see the need for a sustained response to the HIV/AIDS threat, and condom use had its appeal, but through the logic of women's self-protection. So, we took up condoms as the first step in empowering the group. The immediate need was to build capacity among the women for their own self-protection and client education.

The process began with the selection of peer educators who lived in close proximity to those they were educating. The premise was that insiders are more effective than outsiders in reaching the community. Starting from a mere 15 peer educators for 260 women in Gokul Nagar, the peer education programme today is spread over half a dozen districts, where 120 women distribute 350,000 condoms to 5,000 women in prostitution and sex work each month. The programme covers a wide range of locations: women in prostitution and sex work walking the streets, operating in shanty colonies such as Gokul Nagar, doing sex work at industrial sites, lodges, commercial eating and resting places on inter-city roads and national highways. When the programme first began there was one peer educator for seven houses in a row in Gokul Nagar; a group of women living in a cluster chose one from among themselves to be a peer educator. Now, with the spread of awareness, one peer educator caters to up to 40 women.

The peer educators of SANGRAM are trained over a one-year period into understanding the basic nature of the epidemic, sexually transmitted infections, their own vulnerability to the infection, and easy methods of self-protection. As neighbour, friend, and fellow from the same trade, the peer educator has a relatively greater influence on those for whom she has assumed charge. Her tasks comprise relentless re-education of her peers to reinforce the understanding of the condom as a measure of protection, and ensuring that they are in possession of condoms at all times. She must do the following: procure condoms through government agencies that offer them free of cost, distribute them among the women and girls in her jurisdiction, stress the need to keep condoms handy at all times and, under no circumstances, to succumb to a client who refuses to use a condom; train and counsel women who are still undecided about condom use and, provide access to reliable health care services for those who have a sexually transmitted infection or any other health problem.

Looking back, I realise how very slowly and painfully the peer education programme gathered momentum. I had also begun to realise that my own understanding of these women was still woefully inadequate. I had started out under the mistaken impression that there existed a cohesive community of women in prostitution with well-defined common interests. In reality, what I was discovering was that for the women to connect with one another within the brothel situation was a hugely difficult challenge. They were acutely distrustful of each other and competed to woo and retain clients. A deep-rooted feeling of insecurity came in the way of common commitment to self-protection through condom use. In the early stages of the programme, the peer educators found themselves spurned, and even the majority of the women accepting the condom supplies simply did not use them. The biggest stumbling block was the fear of losing a client, the fear that condom enforcement would result in his moving on to someone else who did not lay down such a precondition.

Collective discussion and self-evaluation

It became clear that we had to change our approach, from one of targeting individual women in prostitution and sex work to one of raising collective consciousness. Any viable strategy had to take into account the sex workers' interaction with each other as well as their interaction with the client. Since there was no question of my watching how they entertained their clients, nor could I fathom their inner feelings of competition and camaraderie within the group, I realised that we had to create group situations within which women could give voice to individual as well as common concerns, doubts and fears.

By now, I had become an unavoidable accessory in the life of this community, and they realised that I was there to stay. I started the practice of initiating casual meetings at convenient spots and ordering food and soft drinks for the few women who participated in these chat sessions. Slowly the numbers increased and we found ourselves moving into discussions of serious issues that worried the women: violence, self-respect, dignity, HIV/AIDS and the growing epidemic. Before we realised it we found ourselves doing strategy planning in a collective mode. The question to which we returned again and again was: how could a community such as this consolidate itself and interact with both clients and the outside world without fear? As the discussions grew more intense I proposed that we introduce an element of fun into these meetings. The response was enthusiastic and together we came up with the plan of putting up skits and plays where some of those present would do role playing: some would act as clients, others as authoritarian *gharwalis*, yet others as *maalaks* (stable clients whom women in prostitution and sex work take as paramours and for whom they have the same reverence and respect that normally married women are supposed to have for their husbands). Notions of good and evil surfaced: for example, why is the label of 'evil person' or 'person of easy virtue' used only with reference to women in prostitution and sex work while male clients who visit brothels face no threats to their reputation? Again, women were becoming aware that the HIV virus might be creeping into their midst, and questions about how the virus is contracted, what preventive actions can be taken, began to be openly raised and discussed in the group meetings. The relevance of condom use was now beginning to be understood. Over time, this has become a non-negotiable issue in their sexual practice, and today a client would be hard put to find a sex worker in this community willing to have sex without the protection of a condom.

However, the building of a collective consciousness where knowledge is open and shared had its own backlash. The woman who had opened the gates to the community for me, and who was the first role model for the new organisation – Aprava *mausi* – had a young daughter in sex work. The girl began to noticeably fall sick at frequent intervals, and with their new-found awareness about HIV/AIDS, the women in the community quickly deduced that she was infected. Reacting with feelings of acute aversion, they began to avoid contact with the family. Then, another girl fell victim, and unable to bear the ensuing stigma she drowned herself in a nearby lake.

The suicide disturbed the sense of complacency within the community. Angry mutterings and feelings of discontent began to surface. Some said that the frequent and open discussions about the disease had created a phobia about it of which the suicide was a reflection. Some expressed cynicism about the prevention campaign against HIV/AIDS, and doubted that the solutions and methods being advocated had any efficacy. A sense of being at siege, and fears of becoming further stigmatised by mainstream society and even within their own community due to the HIV epidemic took over the community. The women began to suspect that all this talk about prevention through condom use was a ploy to make them submit to HIV testing in order to serve some selfish agenda of powerful forces within the larger society.

Through all this feeling of disquiet, more and more women in the community began to fall repeatedly sick. Most were diagnosed with TB. But the treatment that they took for it gave them little relief. After several episodes of prolonged illness, these women agreed to be tested for HIV. They tested positive. Regular clients – a major source of income and emotional ties – were also testing positive.

This proved to be the turning point for the condoms-as-a-self-protective-tool campaign. It also forcefully brought to the fore the imperative of collective action if the women were to lead a life of dignity within the community and in relation to the outside world.

Ill health has deep economic and emotional implications for women in prostitution. Their poverty compels the women to work every single day, and when already meagre earnings disappear into medication, frustration begins to run high. For women who test positive fears about their own future and the future of their children deepen, and the loss of regular clients – virtual members of the family – exacerbates the sense of desolation. The presence of SANGRAM in their midst seemed to offer to these women an alternative to retreating into individual grief, fear and inaction.

New directions: Establishing a collective of women in prostitution and sex work

SANGRAM and VAMP

From this followed the next step, the establishment of a new registered collective with the aim of consolidating a common identity among the women and empowering them to find their own solutions. SANGRAM had been initiated and fostered by a middle class activist, backed by a Board of Trustees also from the middle class. The new organisation, although initiated by SANGRAM, would be exclusively a collective of women in prostitution and sex work with its own Board. It would be called Veshya

AIDS Mukabla Parishad (VAMP), roughly translated as 'collective of women in prostitution and sex work to combat AIDS'.

The organisation would be an innovation of sorts, there being no precedent of a formally registered collective of women in prostitution and sex work in the country. Sex work is not a legally recognised activity in India; the law prohibits soliciting or the running of a brothel, but is silent on prostitution *per se*. Thus, the organisation did not fit the stereotype of registered bodies of workers such as trade unions, nor did it have any resemblance to charities or NGOs, i.e., other actors with a similar mission in the public/AIDS arena. It was necessary to take a sound legal opinion on the matter.

More important, it was necessary to get further confirmation from the sex workers themselves that they were indeed keen on forming such a collective. At a camp organised in March 1995 at Ganapatipule, a seaside resort on the Konkan coast also famous as a place of pilgrimage to the Hindu god Ganesha worshipped as the 'Remover of All Obstacles', over 150 women in prostitution and sex work assembled at the invitation of SANGRAM. A lawyer, reputed for taking up public causes and known for his sympathy for disadvantaged groups, was also invited. A detailed questionnaire prepared by Dr. Vijay Thakur – our long time advisor – was administered to the women present to gauge their commitment to the proposal. Their verdict was overwhelmingly positive and in favour of a registered, volunteer-based, non-governmental organisation. All agreed that the principal concern of VAMP should be the AIDS virus, since it posed such a huge threat to their very lives. The Hindi word '*mukabla*' – 'to combat' – in the name of the proposed organisation, was meant to project the strategy of the collective. On the flip side, the acronym VAMP appealed to the women, as the role of the vamp in Indian cinema amused them. For many women in prostitution and sex work the vamp in Indian cinema was a kindred soul, much maligned with nobody bothering to enquire into or understand the compulsions of her life circumstances.

The lawyer assured the group of the legal soundness of their proposal and offered his professional services free of cost to get the proposed collective registered. He was assigned the responsibility of preparing the requisite legal documents such as the Memorandum of Association and the rules and regulations that would govern the functioning of the collective. A Governing Body from among the women themselves was constituted, and an application was made to the Registrar's office to formally register the collective as a legal entity. The Registrar rejected the application on the grounds that the association did not fall within the range of associations that had been granted recognition hitherto. But the persistence of the group's legal advisor who argued that sex workers had a right to come together for their own welfare, helped gain approval for the body in 1996 from the Registrar of Societies for the State of Maharashtra. This was the group's first taste of victory.

At the very outset, the Trustees of SANGRAM (myself included) had made it clear that one of the conditions of VAMP's birth was that ultimately VAMP would have to sustain itself on its own, and that SANGRAM would play only a catalytic role. Among the most crucial resources for any sustained activity are finances and managerial skills. SANGRAM's role would be to provide and mobilise these inputs for VAMP's initial activities. For me as the founder of SANGRAM, this was the beginning of what I foresaw as a dialectical process. SANGRAM had emerged to begin a process of empowerment of a severely disadvantaged community of women – women in prostitution and sex work – in Sangli district. The process had flowered into the establishment of a new organisation which could truly be described as a collective of women in prostitution and sex work, by the women and for the women. The next logical and desirable step must be the completion of the process, i.e., rendering the parent body SANGRAM redundant to the point of its demise as if SANGRAM had willed its own end to happen the moment the purpose of its birth was fulfilled. The sober truth, I knew, was that this accomplishment would depend on how successful VAMP became, and how soon this happened.

VAMP started life with the help of seed money provided by SANGRAM. SANGRAM also helped create a corpus, which has increased in size over the last few years. The team at SANGRAM wrote proposals on VAMP's behalf to seek funding from a few donors. Fortunately by this time, money for AIDS prevention work had begun to flow in through various channels, and VAMP was able to ride this wave with SANGRAM's help. Action Aid was the first agency that vested its trust in VAMP. SANGRAM also provided the secretarial support, managed the accounts, and guided the infant organisation when it launched its community level work.

The HIV/AIDS prevention and control programme of the Government of Maharashtra at the level of each district proved to be a readymade opportunity for VAMP to plunge into action at the level of its own community. There were many features about the government programme that commended it in the eyes of VAMP. It fitted perfectly with VAMP's own principal objective, i.e., combating the HIV virus. For VAMP, its acceptance within the framework of a governmental programme of national importance conferred legitimacy on the organisation vis-à-vis the outside world. And, the spread of the programme across the state's several districts offered opportunities for VAMP to extend its own reach and develop links with distant but culturally related communities of women in prostitution and sex work.

A major component of the government programme is the distribution of condoms free of cost. VAMP volunteers collect the required number of condoms from the district headquarters and distribute them among the women in prostitution and sex work in towns and villages. The distribution itself is organised on a three-tier basis. A field worker indents and collects the condoms from the district headquarters and hands over the required supplies to the community workers who form the second tier. They in turn coordinate with the third tier, the '*tai*' ('sister') who delivers the condoms to the individual women in the community. The common thread that binds them all is the requirement of maintaining a continuous supply of condoms. As of now VAMP has a branch in each of the two districts of Sangli and Solapur to facilitate its work.

Another component of the government programme is the control of sexually transmitted infections (STIs). The VAMP field worker is responsible for identifying STIs and HIV among her constituency. The community worker then lends support in accessing the available government health facilities and, in the case of a woman testing positive, counsels the friends and relatives who are looking after her. The *tai* strives to create empathy and support for the HIV positive woman within the locality.

Setbacks to progress

A drawback of VAMP's identification with the government programme as a vehicle for its own mission has been the obsession of the programme with condom distribution. Admittedly, chanelling all energies into universalising condom use has its plus points. Most importantly, it has taught VAMP activists the art of turning things around to their own advantage. However, it resulted in the relegation of all other aspects of collective empowerment to the sidelines, due to its taking away time from other advocacy and community mobilisation activities with their benefits for VAMP's own internal dynamics and long-term growth prospects.

The involvement in the government programme also threw up the unforeseen challenge of having to re-order mutual expectations between VAMP and other actors in the district, and this generated its own conflicts. The then chief government functionary in the district administration resented SANGRAM's highly proactive role through the agency of VAMP volunteers. As a bureaucrat, he had the characteristic air of condescension towards all those below him in the social and official hierarchy, and expected a patron-client equation with those who came forward to associate themselves with the government in any capacity. He was not prepared for the SANGRAM-led VAMP team, which did not see itself as anybody's client, and which went about its HIV/AIDS prevention and control work with a missionary zeal. This inevitably led to friction. Another source of conflict came from a petty politician in the district who saw

SANGRAM as a threat to his own hold over the community of women in prostitution and sex work. He went on to activate the familiar *'babu-neta'* ('government functionary-politician') nexus, resulting in an attempt by the combined efforts of these two men to terminate VAMP's involvement in the government programme and thus marginalise SANGRAM. VAMP's cadres of volunteers were lured to leave VAMP and join the government's component of the programme, with a view to create disarray and demoralisation in the NGO's ranks.

These damaging tactics were initially successful. VAMP's work came to a temporary halt, and several of its workers permitted themselves to be poached by the government programme. However, other unfolding processes intervened to stall this turn of events. In the course of a routine administrative shuffle, the hostile bureaucrat was promoted and his successor saw the futility of his predecessor's attempt to get the government to take over a task that was being admirably discharged by an NGO. Nor did he sympathise with the politician who was trying to erode SANGRAM's influence within the sex worker community. Further, the volunteers who had left SANGRAM began to return for their own reasons. The top-down administrative structure within the government with its rigid hierarchy, where the field worker – the point of contact – is the least valued rung, was a far cry from the autonomy, initiative, mutual responsibility and dignity that had characterised the volunteers' experience of their roles within the SANGRAM-VAMP-run programme. In a sense, loyalty to SANGRAM and support to VAMP came back on the rebound, as the volunteers who returned after a brief spell with the government-run programme went on to become the most committed workers in the organisation. It was their enthusiasm for enhancing their own skills and efficiency in the interests of VAMP's greater effectiveness that led to a new round of training for the volunteers. Again, it was SANGRAM that arranged for this training. At a four-day camp, volunteers were trained in the issues of HIV testing, care of positive patients, managing doctor-patient interaction, and dealing with violence and police harassment.

Hard won gains

Over time, the combined efforts of SANGRAM and VAMP have reaped many successes. They have effectively raised the level of demand for better quality condoms within the government's district level programme. Civil surgeons in government-run district hospitals in the region are being made to feel accountable to sex worker patients, and some hospitals in the district have even been persuaded to change their timings for case paper submissions to suit the unusually late hours kept by women in prostitution. Work has also been ongoing with the police to bring home to them the futility of raiding and harassing women who work in brothels. Most significantly, women in prostitution are beginning to understand the need for a collective voice, and are beginning to demand it. They now have the self-esteem to reveal who they are, free from any sense of shame. VAMP also issues identity cards to its peer educators to facilitate their access to hospitals when taking fellow women for testing and treatment for STIs; these educators are trained in the recognition of STI symptoms and understanding hospital administrative procedures. Almost all of them say that they are proud to be card-holding members of their own collective organisation. This pride in being open about who they are acts as a role model for their sisters in prostitution.

The condom distribution programme has also been effective. The women began to experience a drop in sexually transmitted infections, and suddenly saw that their health was improving. In several areas where sex work is concentrated, there is now 100 per cent condom usage across brothels, and those clients who refuse to comply are turned away. In other areas, peer educators strive to arrive at this level of self-confidence among women in prostitution and sex work. "We want business, but we don't want AIDS", is the women's refrain.

Condom use enforcement, as stressed by the peer educators, works in many ways. It can be truly achieved only if each and every woman in a community agrees to do so, building on the norm of never losing a client, and keeping the collective interest in mind. If every woman enforces condom use, all the women will stay healthy and can continue to work, even in the time of HIV. This holds true for independent women in prostitution and sex work and for *gharwalis* who run brothels. Further, condom use by all obviates any pernicious distinction between women who are healthy and women who are positive. Among these women there is an unspoken rule: nobody ever asks which woman has tested positive. Admitting that one is positive is like a death sentence for a woman whose survival depends on selling sex.

The condom distribution programme has also had a broader impact in terms of HIV/AIDS prevention. Enforcing condom use with a client means explaining why he must wear the condom. This creates a chain of information that is vital to prevent the spread of HIV, and sets into motion long-term changes in male sexual behaviour. As VAMP activists say they explain to clients who insist that they want the 'fun' of 'body on body'. "The fun is only for two minutes, but if you use a condom you can enjoy the rest of your life. If your two minutes of pleasure is reduced by 5 per cent, what is the big deal?"

The development of skills for home-based care of positive women led by peers has been another gain. Peers have become de-facto caregivers of women who fall sick, caring for their children and even their sick lovers in their absence, arranging for funerals of women who die, and supporting women and their families through their most painful moments.

From women in prostitution and sex work to the wider society: Expanding SANGRAM's reach

Clients of women in prostitution and sex work are only the tip of the proverbial iceberg. They are windows to the predominantly heterosexual community in the wider society where universal marriage is the norm. Married men and unmarried adolescents who visit women in prostitution and sex work both go back to unsuspecting wives/brides in marital unions. Against this backdrop, a peer education programme that restricts itself to women in prostitution is limited in reach. As VAMP's active members say, "If we really want to stem the tide, we have to build dams at different bends in the river." SANGRAM believes that when it comes to HIV, a woman in prostitution and a married woman are like two sides of the same coin, since both are at equal risk of getting HIV from the same man. However, unlike the former, the latter does not realise that she is sexually at risk of HIV since she believes that she is in a monogamous relationship.

In 1997, with VAMP having been put on its way to relative autonomy, SANGRAM was able to turn its attention to designing programmes – called the District Campaign – to include the larger community, especially married women living with their husbands. From the outset, and beginning with Sangli district, its focus was to be on three constituents: rural household women who have no access to knowledge of HIV and who are vulnerable due to their husbands' irresponsible behaviour; young adults who are mobile, growing into independence, and who need information, education and counselling on issues of sexual health and sexual and gender rights; and male adolescents, who constitute a considerable proportion of the clients of women in prostitution and sex work, who refuse to use condoms, and show up significantly as HIV positive cases in Sangli's Civil Hospital. Today, the District Campaign covers over 713 villages.

It was not easy to recruit female social workers to travel in the villages for the District Campaign. For one, women do not take up travelling jobs that require leaving home overnight, and additionally there was the stigma attached to HIV and sexuality-related work. SANGRAM found a way out by adopting a policy of positive discrimination, i.e., recruiting and training widows, deserted women, and lower caste women who had fewer restrictions on their movements, who needed the jobs and who, like women in prostitution and sex work, were marginalised people who needed to be empowered. Joined by male social workers, these women build rapport with household women in villages and gather social data about each village as a means of building village level support.

However, for the rural married women whom SANGRAM's workers are trying to reach out to, opening themselves up to talking about sex does not come easily. The campaign thus has a component of *maitrin* or girl friend. In every village community the social workers try to identify women who can take on the role of a friend, someone with whom neighbourhood women can discuss intimate matters, often their own extreme vulnerability within marriages where they have no control over their own lives or the means to protect themselves from ill health.

When trying to reach out to young boys and girls, the project found that the urban middle class erected barriers to communication. Most school and college principals in towns believed that the middle class is safe from AIDS, and that the dose of AIDS education that the government had put out to school and college students was more than enough. Principals of rural educational institutions, however, were more receptive. With its approach of a holistic sexuality and gender education, SANGRAM has been working with these students on raising awareness of a wide range of sexuality and gender issues. This activity has also been a route for recruiting a cadre of youth volunteers in a War Against the Spread of AIDS as part of its District Campaign, that includes street plays that often use familiar folk and religious forms and idioms and visual communication through posters and leaflets aimed at adults and youth in the community at large.

Looking back, looking ahead

We could say with some confidence that the process of empowerment has begun among the community of women in prostitution and sex work that SANGRAM is working with. It is a fragile beginning, and it is difficult to predict its course. Will it flounder? Or will it gain in strength? Only time can tell. There are some areas, like violence and other violations of civil rights, where we only continue to firefight. VAMP has made progress in making common cause with other groups similarly disadvantaged, marginalised and stigmatised: women in prostitution and sex work in other states, women who are the victims of violence, people of alternative sexualities, and other sexual minorities. As part of the National Network of Sex Workers, VAMP members are slowly building a common identity with other women in prostitution, and beginning to place their own demands – primarily for decriminalisation of prostitution – on policy platforms. The process of empowerment has built some natural leaders, but they continue to need nurturing, particularly when setbacks occur such as violent attacks on their civil rights by the police often in collusion with local elites. Some capacity-building has taken place for HIV/AIDS prevention and control, and condom use has gained almost universal acceptance among women in prostitution and sex work. This is likely to stay unless some exogenous factor dictates otherwise at a later date. As for fellowship, cooperation and collective action, we have not struck any deep roots yet. In this tentative equilibrium, any kind of imbalance can occur at any point in time.

According to my own test of its success, VAMP's viability would become a fact only when I as an individual and the entity of SANGRAM as a catalyst cease to be relevant to its existence. As of now, we continue to remain central to the momentum and sustenance of the process described in this chapter. If anything, at the present time, not just I but also my entire family are engulfed in the daily turmoil of VAMP's self-creation. My journalist husband is almost always co-opted in case of a crisis and we get emotionally drawn into all the processes of VAMP. This is not a complaint, nor a martyr's lament. The cause of women in prostitution and sex work is still one deserving of our total devotion. And I am confident that my redundancy would come about sooner or later. About SANGRAM's future, I am not in a position to predict, but I remain hopeful for VAMP.

SECTION FIVE

HIV/AIDS as a Human Rights Issue and Men Who Have Sex with Men

An Overview

Several people within the health sector ask what is all this new noise being made about the treatment rights of people with HIV/AIDS, when millions of adults and children in this country are suffering and dying of poverty-related diseases with no effective rights to prevention and cure. What about *their* human rights to health, they ask. Some question the wisdom of government spending its scarce resources on a life-long treatment with expensive anti-retroviral drugs for all positive people simply because it is a human rights requirement. Within the health care sector, doctors and other staff question the rights of people with HIV/AIDS to expect medical treatment ~nd even equality with other sick people when they themselves are 'responsible' for their plight due to their 'immoral' sexual behaviour. But by far the severest societal stigma in the context of HIV is reserved for women in prostitution and those believed to engage in 'unnatural' sexual behaviours, – men who have sex with men (MSM) and other persons of alternative sexual orientations – who are seen to be violating society's norm of heterosexuality as the only natural form of sexual behaviour.

When we speak of HIV/AIDS as a human rights issue, we invoke the rights to life, liberty and employment free of discrimination as guaranteed in the Indian Constitution, and to the rights to health and sexual choice as guaranteed in international social and economic covenants. What this means is that in the eyes of the law, all citizens have the right to knowledge, information and available practical means to protect themselves from HIV infection. And, if infected due to ignorance or negligence, have the right to fair and just treatment in medical establishments, non-discriminatory treatment in their place of work, and the right to residence in their communities without harassment.

The above framework applies generally to all persons. However, there are some sections of society that are particularly disenfranchised with relation to HIV, such as men who have sex with men (MSM). The pre-existing stigmatisation and isolation of MSM from the mainstream acquires greater poignancy in the context of HIV, since they cannot even talk about their lives and sexual orientation openly for fear of social prejudice, and because they lack strong bonds of community for self help unlike even sex workers.

In India, Section 377 of the Indian Penal Code (IPC) framed in 1860 criminalises as "unnatural" those who do not conform to the dominant norm of heterosexuality. It states that "whosoever has carnal intercourse voluntarily against the order of nature with any man, woman or animal shall be punished with imprisonment for life, or imprisonment for a term which may extend to 10 years, and shall be liable to fine". Beat police encountering a person or persons whose sexual orientation they decide is suspect, feel free to threaten to charge them under Section 377, and sexually violate them as their own form of 'punishment', or otherwise harass or torture them or extort money, even when circumstances are not incriminating under the law. Fear of disclosure of their sexual orientation and the implications of this for their family or employment status deter most MSM from raising their voices in protest or publicising this violation of their citizenship rights.

One of the unprecedented outcomes of HIV in India is that it has propelled MSM into visibility. In the process it has highlighted the extreme vulnerability of MSM to both HIV and to hate crimes. MSM tend to suffer in many ways: a low sense of self-esteem, psychological confusion regarding their sexual orientation, and a primary and secondary socialisation experience marked by harassment and ridicule for their, often, different mannerisms and traits, i.e., nonconformity to societal norms of masculinity. They also lack the comfort of an alternative set of socially accepted norms and behaviours, with the attendant organisational supports to help them deal with psychological and physical assaults from the heterosexual majority population. Both these sets of factors result in most adult MSM being forced into marriage by families keen to conform to the cultural norm of universal marriage. On the part of MSM themselves, the desperate desire to conform to norms of 'normalcy' and familial duties, as well as the social advantage accruing to marriage versus having to combat the stigma of being single or being open about their alternative sexuality, lead them to resort to marriage as a means of buying peace, after which they carry on with their MSM sexual activity secretly. Many others marry with the hope of thereby being 'cured' of their 'disease'. Once married, social pressures upon them continue: to sexually relate to their wives and produce children – particularly male children – as symbols of their masculinity. The routes of HIV transmission are, therefore, considerably interlinked, involving MSM, women and children.

Although impossible to estimate, there are believed to be around 50 million MSM in India. Apart from a handful of NGOs working with MSMs there are virtually no ongoing sexual health interventions for this vulnerable group. The overall insensitivity to the needs of this group – whether in government HIV policies and programmes, the private medical community, the media, or even among NGOs working in reproductive health –, makes it difficult for them to access reliable information and referrals through any of these sources.

MSM vulnerability to HIV rests on several factors. Physiologically, penetrative anal sex is riskier in terms of transmission of HIV infection than penile-vaginal sex, due to the high possibility of rupture of membranes and bleeding in the anal area, which facilitates the entry of the virus if either partner is already infected. If either of the partners already has some other sexually transmitted infection (STI), HIV transmission again becomes easier, as the lesions caused by the STI facilitate the entry of the HIV virus. Sexually transmitted infections among MSM often remain untreated due to MSM fears of approaching mainstream doctors who may judge them unfavourably, humiliate or even reject them. And untreated STIs are a major risk factor for HIV transmission among men, as among women.

Other social factors operate as well. MSM generally lack information and education on how to understand their sexual orientation and its implications for their personal and social life. There is also the misconception that HIV is transmitted only through vaginal sex and that anal sex is safe, since heterosexuality is assumed to be universal and all public messages about HIV/AIDS refer to heterosexual sex. The lack of privacy for MSM sexual activity means that the sex act is most often hurriedly carried out in public spaces such as urinals and parks. Hence, even for those MSM who are aware of condoms as a protective device, time and space constraints make it difficult to negotiate safe sex. Several MSM who have practised unsafe sex are fearful of approaching health care services lest their sexual behaviour become public and they be treated as unnatural, criminal and HIV positive, a triple stigma. Confidentiality issues around HIV testing in India are still problematic, and there are no unambiguous guidelines for doctors and nurses on how to treat people with HIV, particularly if the patient also happens to be an MSM; this further alienates potential MSM patients from mainstream medical services. Ironically, most mainstream health services assume that people are heterosexual. When they record a patient's age, income and profession, they rarely ask for the person's sexual orientation. As a result, there is little real Indian data that can help us understand the journey of the epidemic within the Indian MSM community. Where MSM have received social visibility it has been negative, in the form of haphazard or sensational media reporting. Generally, these have followed on controversies such as the arrest of MSM activists merely because they were distributing condoms and sexuality/ AIDS-related literature as part of their voluntary work as

HIV/AIDS activists. This is dubbed by the police as criminal activity, i.e., soliciting, and being in possession of pornographic literature.

The chapter that follows on the Naz Foundation's work helps unravel the situation of MSM, and presents the process of capacity-building for this group that the Naz Foundation steers. Naz is one of the leading pioneers in the country in its innovative combination of advocacy and service efforts in the cause of HIV prevention in the general population and among MSM in particular. In the nearly ten years of Naz's existence, the situation has changed for the MSM community in many far-reaching ways. Support groups for Hindi and English language speaking MSM, telephone help lines, educational and training manuals, testing and treatment services have all come into existence, albeit mainly in metropolitan cities. The numbers using these services have grown steadily, and there is also a growing sense of community and a maturing of self-confidence and autonomy in the ability to deal with law and order agencies that continue to view them as deviants.

Networking has also been afoot among MSM groups in different parts of the country, many of which have been able to come into existence due to efforts of leaders in the field such as Naz and Humsafar (another group based in Mumbai). Their dream is for a more just and equitable society that respects diversity, including sexual diversity. One of the strengths driving these groups is the commitment of its members to activism. Groups like Naz have played an invaluable role in providing their volunteers and full-time programme personnel with the opportunity and challenge to initiate new programmes, and the flexibility to take these initiatives in different directions. For those with long-term involvement with Naz, work may be as varied and enriching as doing counselling; helping start support groups in other parts of the country; carrying out research and documentation; participating in local, national and international conferences; preparing manuals on sexuality for MSM; participating in *dharnas* (pickets) to protest against persecution of individuals; doing case by case advocacy with the National

Human Rights Commission; or lobbying for repeal of Section 377. Networking has also encompassed working with other NGOs – in the field of feminist rights, women's reproductive health, or sex workers' rights – to help them integrate an MSM perspective (and concerns) into their work.

The chapter also highlights how advocacy in the absence of service back up lacks substance. HIV education among vulnerable groups is creating a demand for testing and treatment services, but the failure of the mainstream medical profession to respond to the HIV/AIDS epidemic is compelling NGOs to set up such services. Hence, a lot of Naz's awareness-raising work tries to reach out to the medical profession. Naz's experience also demonstrates how NGOs are inevitably drawn into further and ever further expansion. Provision of services, for example, cannot be confined to any single targeted group. When a service treats one section of stigmatised people – in this case MSM – with dignity and respect and shows them a way forward, it is inevitable that persons from other stigmatised groups across the social spectrum, i.e., HIV positive people in general and positive women in particular, also begin flocking to it, challenging it to expand its scope. Nor can services end with the clinic. The social rehabilitation of positive persons within their households and communities of residence, and economic rehabilitation of people in advancing stages of the disease continues to be a major challenge.

Client Advocacy and Service Provision
The Naz Foundation's Mission

ANJALI GOPALAN

The issue of HIV/AIDS goes beyond its identity as an infectious disease. It is deeply personal in so far as it is linked to sex and sexuality, both taboo subjects in India. It is also a minefield of misinformation, something that leads inevitably to a climate of fear, discrimination and human rights abuses.

Naz came into existence in 1994, at a time when the HIV/AIDS epidemic was just unfolding in India. Its mission was first and foremost to advocate the human rights of people in relation to HIV/AIDS. This involved both direct advocacy at an individual personal level, and indirect advocacy through the dissemination of information, training, education, and negotiation with other groups concerned with the HIV/AIDS epidemic. Simultaneously, it was committed to providing HIV/AIDS-related services. The struggle to maintain a creative tension – or balance – between the two roles of advocacy and service provision has characterised Naz's evolution and growth.

As the founder of Naz, it was inevitable that my understanding and experience would colour the mission objectives of the organisation. My own previous background of work in HIV/AIDS had been in the U.S. in the 1980s, during the early days of the epidemic in that country. I was familiar with the literature and techniques of advocacy and awareness raising. My experience also included working with gay men in the U.S., the community that was the first to be visibly struck down by the virus. One lesson that I had learnt was the crucial importance of complementing service provision with advocacy work. In India of the early 1990s, where HIV/AIDS was just beginning to be acknowledged as a mainstream problem, this had even greater relevance. For Naz to simply 'provide a service', under these conditions, seemed unrealistic. Without the broad-based advocacy required to maintain the service and make it accessible (and known) to the people who needed it, a service organisation could well find itself in a situation of eroding relevance due to disuse of the service. Conversely, if Naz were to focus solely on advocating for rights, without the back-up of services to meet the needs and demands of people with HIV/AIDS, i.e., give concrete substance to their rights after having raised their awareness of these rights, its advocacy work would remain hollow and unsustainable.

The initial years

At the time that Naz came into existence, our aim was a modest one, i.e., to go some way toward filling a gap in both information and services available in the country in the area of HIV/AIDS. At the time, there were few programmes and initiatives in operation. The first reported case of AIDS in India had been in 1986, and for the next few years very little had been attempted in the country by way of recognising the significance and magnitude of the problem, and devising strategies to counter the onslaught of the coming epidemic. The rate of infection was rising steadily, but official attitudes as well as general public opinion was one of complacency. The common perception was that the disease had perhaps come to India, but there was no cause for worry. It was 'something that happened to other people', people lacking in 'morals', people who were not worth worrying about.

The scene in 1994 was one of ignorance and indifference all around. HIV was perceived as a health problem, but the public health machinery was inert. To begin with, even within the medical community many were not adequately informed about

HIV/AIDS. Their knowledge was often inaccurate and incomplete, and the fact that many of them were uncomfortable with working around issues of sex and sexuality acted as an effective barrier to self-improvement. Linked to this was the fact that the public awareness programmes that existed were often rooted in unrealistic understanding of social, sexual and personal realities. Very little was known about actual risk behaviours and the factors that shaped these behaviours. Intervention programmes therefore tended to focus on just a few groups considered to be at 'high risk', such as truck drivers or commercial sex workers. Undoubtedly, both these groups needed immediate attention, as they were indeed greatly vulnerable to the infection. But the trumpeting of the HIV/AIDS prevention programme as a programme for high-risk groups carried the risk of equating HIV/AIDS exclusively with these groups, and devalued its grave significance for the entire society. It bolstered the commonly held view that HIV happened only to people with 'loose' morals, and that it could not filter into mainstream society, which was perceived as upholding the Indian cultural values of monogamy and mutual fidelity on the part of all those bound in matrimony.

Not since the advent of leprosy has such a culture of discrimination afflicted the victims of a disease as has happened in the case of HIV/AIDS. As with leprosy, the fear associated with HIV/AIDS is not only because it is an infectious disease but also because of the social stigma attached. Most people know that HIV can be transmitted from one human being to another; however, they lack in precise understanding of how this transmission takes place. Even more than in the case of leprosy, myth, mystery and misunderstanding surround the modes of transmission of the HIV virus. Inaccurate or wrong information leads to false beliefs, which in turn lead to targeting of and discrimination against certain groups or individuals. Naz from the start consciously took upon itself the task of debunking myths regarding the transmission of HIV, since discriminatory treatment on the grounds of HIV/AIDS is a violation of human rights. This stress on HIV/AIDS as a human rights issue has been integral to all its training and educational sessions.

Among its earliest activities, therefore, were the dissemination of correct information and the launching of a series of training programmes. In this Naz threw its net wide to include a vast range of audiences: health care professionals; NGOs, particularly those working on women's issues; youth groups, particularly students coming to terms with their sexuality; and, men who have sex with men (MSM), a totally invisible sexual sub-culture until Naz identified itself with them. For all of the above-mentioned groups, Naz was one of the earliest NGOs that brought HIV/AIDS up close to their line of vision. But in relation to MSM – particularly in its exploration into strategies appropriate to their needs as a high-risk group – Naz was virtually the sole pioneer. Although we commenced our work with advocacy, it soon became obvious that this absolutely had to be backed up with services to match. A major concern that was voiced again and again in the course of the training sessions was the near-total absence of any support services in relation to HIV prevention, testing or care. Similarly, the awareness-raising work with the MSM community brought to the fore the demand for counselling, testing and treatment services specifically sensitive to their needs.

In the absence of appropriate services, Naz's response to this yawning gap was to begin providing the various services itself. These soon included women's and men's sexual health programmes, outreach to communities such as street children and, eventually, counselling, care and support around HIV/AIDS itself. These programmes have been expanding ever since. Today, a care home for destitute HIV positive adults and orphaned children, and medical, counselling and nutritional services for home-based treatment and care of positive persons in poor communities in Delhi, are among Naz's extensive activities. The next step envisioned is the rehabilitation of positive persons within their own communities, through fostering (often new) skills and creating income-earning opportunities within families where the main breadwinners are afflicted with HIV.

Training workshops

Sensitising and training the medical community into the complex issues surrounding HIV was among the early initiatives of Naz. Naz had observed that while misinformation among the general public was common, many professionals in the medical and health communities were as misinformed as lay people. While most doctors seemed to have a good grasp of the facts surrounding the virus itself, some of their views – that HIV is connected with 'loose morals', that high risk persons should be compulsorily tested and segregated in order to 'protect' society – revealed complete insensitivity to the human rights of those involved, views that were antithetical to the values and beliefs that Naz upheld.

In 1997, Naz carried out a Knowledge, Attitudes and Practices (KAP) survey of 32 medical interns in a leading teaching hospital in New Delhi. Shockingly, over half the interns believed that the disease was a threat to India due to the vitiating impact on people's morals of 'Western lifestyles and values', and that the way to prevent the spread of HIV was by promoting 'Indian values'. While they all agreed that counselling was important both before and after an HIV test, they held on to stereotypes regarding who ought to be tested. Over 80 per cent of the respondents supported compulsory testing for sex workers and drug users. TB patients and street children were next on their list of those requiring surveillance. Contrary to the stipulation of the government's National AIDS Control Organisation (NACO) – the agency monitoring the AIDS situation in India –, half the interns participating in the survey were of the opinion that HIV/AIDS patients ought to be segregated in separate wards in hospitals. These results of a survey, albeit small in size, confirmed several casual observations by the Naz team.

This added urgency to Naz's decision to build bridges with hospital-based health personnel, and to work proactively by holding more workshops for them and seek to change this attitude. Naz lobbied hard with the management of city hospitals – public and private – to run these workshops for their staff. The idea was to create a climate for better and more humane treatment of HIV/AIDS patients coming to these hospitals.

But such lobbying has not always been able to overcome resistance. Even when workshops are held, doctors have tended to stay away. And private managements have tended to stress doctors' rights alone, with little willingness to accommodate patients' rights. At the level of support staff, a potent combination of prejudice and infrastructural shortcomings works to stigmatise positive patients. A recurrent complaint of nurses especially in government-run hospitals is that even basic precautionary equipment such as gloves is not available to them. Naz recognises that under such circumstances fear of infection on the part of these support staff is genuine. For this reason Naz supplies protective equipment for the patients it refers to hospitals. Government authorities on their part assert that all government hospital staff *is* provisioned with gloves. This is similar to government assertions that all hospitals are stocked with drugs for opportunistic infections such as TB. Yet, in reality, Naz has found that most often neither of these resources are consistently or universally accessible to those who need them, whether patients or support staff. This compromises the rights of both patients and providers. Balancing the rights of patients with those of medical and health professionals is an issue that can be tackled only through collaboration between different arms of civil society. This requires strong efforts in advocacy, advocacy that includes accountability of public as well as private institutions to the general population and to the rights of HIV/AIDS patients in particular.

The recent availability of anti-retroviral (ARV) drugs has had a significant impact on the treatment scenario, some of which is worrisome. It has posed new challenges to Naz in its advocacy and training work with medical professionals. In some respects, the medical community has now become more open to entertaining HIV/AIDS patients. But this largely stops with prescribing ARV drugs. Rarely is any consideration given to patients' capacity to afford the treatment in a sustainable manner, which includes not only the cocktail of drugs themselves but also monitoring for reactions and for drug resistance over the long term. Raising awareness among doctors about ARV drugs and treatment regimens is a task that Naz has undertaken recently.

Another activity that has gained in strength over the years are the training courses offered by Naz to NGOs, educational and advocacy groups in civil society, particularly those focusing on women, and international charities and aid agencies that have field offices in India, on how to incorporate HIV/AIDS-related knowledge and practices for prevention and control into their ongoing programmes. Sometimes, the customised training programmes are in response to requests from these organisations themselves. Very often, Naz itself seeks out and lobbies NGOs or NGO networks that it identifies as potentially receptive or having a wide reach, e.g., those with field offices across the country (such as the Family Planning Association of India), or those that send health education trainers to field based NGOs in different parts of the country (such as CHETNA). It also requests donor agencies – such as UNICEF or Oxfam – to recommend their grantee organisations for such training, since the increased inflow of international funds into HIV work has been an important factor in more and more NGOs entering HIV work. What it offers is a full-length training programme over a year, comprising three semesters. The entire training is formulated around the themes of self-evaluation and problem-solving. Participants are encouraged to bring their field experiences into the classroom. This varied material is used to help trainees apply what they are learning, and it has also helped to steadily enrich and diversify the training modules. Training workshops also serve as the most important source of revenue for Naz. It keeps Naz going as a self-sustaining organisation that is not driven by grants alone. It also makes it possible for Naz to pursue its other activities and, particularly in the case of its advocacy work, follow its own independent path of action.

In its early phase, Naz worked intensively with youth, particularly with students. The effort focused mainly on lobbying with school and college managements for introducing sexuality and sexual health education. This is no longer a sustained programme, largely because there are today many more organisations doing sexuality education among urban youth. Also, Naz has been increasingly chanellising its own energies into work with MSM groups, the care home for positive persons, and home-based treatment and care.

Counselling as a tool to empowerment and the dilemma of client confidentiality

While the foregoing account of Naz's advocacy and service activities describes its attempts at creating a positive and respectful social environment for those disadvantaged in relation to the HIV/AIDS epidemic, an important aspect of its work consists in direct advocacy at the individual level. A fundamental principle in Naz's approach is that personalised support programmes are a more effective tool for sustained behaviour change and empowerment than the generalised impersonal approach to awareness raising consisting of posters and leaflets that characterise a large part of HIV/AIDS awareness programmes.

One of the basic premises on which Naz was founded is the empowerment of individual people. It is Naz's philosophy that every person has the right to live the way he or she chooses; accordingly, Naz assists people in the exercise of their lifestyle and sexual choices. In pursuance of this goal, Naz offers a counselling service. It consists of:

— telephone help lines, separately for HIV positive persons, for gay men (Humraz), and for lesbians (Sangini);
— pre- and post-HIV test counselling; and
— counselling for people living with HIV/AIDS (PLWHA) and their families.

In Naz's experience, individual counselling by trained counsellors is one of the most effective tools for empowering the individual. When assured of a safe and confidential environment, people tend to open up with questions and concerns, and real progress can be made in the direction of empowerment through education and support.

Helping an individual along the path of empowerment and autonomous decision-making, however, is fraught with dilemmas. Perhaps the key word for any counsellor the world over is confidentiality. At Naz, this is a crucial policy point, and always takes priority over other concerns. In a field such as HIV/AIDS, this commitment to confidentiality could raise complex challenges. The following case study illustrates this dilemma.

Ram (true name concealed to protect his identity) was a 29-year-old injecting drug user who had tested positive to HIV and started attending counselling sessions at Naz. In the course of the counselling, Ram revealed that he was about to get married very soon. His parents had arranged the marriage with a girl he had never met. Ram was aware of the possibility of infecting the girl if he married her, unless he consistently used condoms during sexual intercourse. Further sessions revealed that Ram had contracted TB and that, in fact, he wanted to get married so he would have someone to take care of him. As the counselling sessions progressed, and a mutual trust grew between Ram and the counsellor, Ram volunteered to postpone the date of his marriage. After a while, Ram revealed that he had begun to frequent commercial sex workers. When asked if he was using condoms, he replied in the negative; his visits to sex workers was usually in a drunken state, and he could not be bothered with condoms. This put the counsellor and others at Naz in a very uncomfortable situation. On the one hand there was this promise to Ram of complete confidentiality about what was shared with the counsellor, while on the other it was a question of protecting the right to informed choice for the person Ram was planning to marry, as well for the commercial sex workers he was visiting and infecting. The fact that practising unsafe sex may have become a habit for Ram during all this time raised the issue of whether he would continue to do this once he was married (although the marriage was postponed, it was not cancelled altogether). Should Ram go ahead with his plan of getting married, at stake was the life of his wife and the lives of the children the couple were likely to have. Ram's behaviour also entailed a chain reaction in spreading the HIV infection. The commercial sex workers he was having sex with surely had other clients as well. Many of them might also be indulging in unprotected sex, thereby endangering themselves and all those they came into sexual contact with, including their spouses. And there was the threat of HIV infection being transmitted to the children born to these couples.

Naz upheld its solemn promise of confidentiality to Ram. One may argue that advocacy on behalf of all these people at risk ought to be a high priority for Naz. Weighed against the notion of service provision (Ram's counselling sessions), the rights of the others to know about his status could be seen as more important for, after all, their lives were at stake. However, the principle of confidentiality is sacred to the organisation.

Naz draws strength from its belief that in the long run personalised support programmes based on trust help people understand the complexity of their situation, and lead them to making considered (and often courageous) choices which would protect their own rights as well as show respect for the rights of others they come into contact with. It is thus a much more effective tool for sustained behaviour change and empowerment, as compared with generalised 'messages' about HIV, fear-inducing exhortations, or didactic/scientific information alone.

Working with men who have sex with men (MSM)

In the context of HIV in India, two groups stand out as the most stigmatised, marginalised and even criminalised. These are sex workers and people of alternative sexualities, the latter most notably men who have sex with men (MSM). Society at large despises them. The communities in whose midst they live reject them. Few NGOs are willing to work with them. And, the government's National AIDS Control Organisation recognises them only as 'target groups' deserving of policy attention, but remains ineffective when other arms of the state such as the police persecute them.

Naz's initiative with MSM was the first ever in the city of Delhi, and among the first in the country. When Naz began its work in 1994, sex among men was not even acknowledged to exist in the public discourse. There was no understanding of the sub-culture, leave alone of how to get HIV/AIDS messages across to them. Given that my background of working with gay communities in the U.S. had already sensitised me to this group, it was inevitable that my circle of acquaintances in Delhi included a number of educated, upper class gay men. Through them I learnt of cruising spots in the city used by local gay men. After a brief survey of these I began to visit one of them, and over a period of time was able to build a rapport with several of the visiting men. I realised that there was a phenomenal amount of MSM sex work going on there, and army personnel from the nearby cantonment dominated the purchaser profile. The majority of the men were already married or would definitely be married soon. They did not see sex between men as sex at all, but as *masti* or fun. And nor did they use condoms; for them condoms were a contraceptive device for use by heterosexual couples alone. It was clear to me that the men's level of comfort with other men was high – possibly fostered by the acute sexual segregation in the Indian cultural context – and that they saw sexual relations between men as just an extension of this interaction. To an AIDS activist, however, the wider repercussions of this were alarming.

Naz swung into action with an outreach programme for condom distribution in these cruising areas. Our simple belief at the time was that direct intervention to promote safer sex was the best option for preventing HIV transmission. However, several months into outreach work, it became apparent that many MSM had greater needs than the safe sex agenda promoted by Naz. The older MSM (*nanis*) resented talk of infection, dismissing it as a 'Western' bogey calculated to bring a halt to sex work. But the younger generation of MSM were full of confusion and anxieties about their sexual identity. They worried about being judged abnormal by others. They agonised that there was no one to whom they could turn for honest advice. They feared that they were 'bad' in some way. The young adults wished for medicines that could stop them being attracted to others of their own sex. The young unmarried men did not know how to resist family pressures on them to marry against their will. Many also expressed fear, ignorance and anxiety about STDs. They were particularly afraid of approaching doctors with problems relating to the anus for fear of rejection.

Clearly, what these young men needed was one-on-one counselling and support. Early in its work, Naz had set up an HIV/AIDS telephone help line service for the general public. This help line had already been reflecting MSM concerns; many callers were asking questions surrounding issues of homosexuality. Naz now launched a set of dedicated help lines specifically for MSM. These were Humraz, an English language help line, and Naz Dost catering to Hindi-speaking MSM.

The help lines proved to be hugely popular and they soon spawned three support groups. Naz itself set up two of these: Humrahi for English speaking gay men, and Humnawaaz for Hindi speaking gay men. Soon, men who frequented MSM sites as *kothis* – passive partners – asked if they could set up their own support group, Humjoli, also under Naz's umbrella, for Hindi speaking *kothis*.

The demand for the above initiatives pointed clearly to one truth. If people have to be taught to protect themselves from HIV, they need first to learn how to value themselves. Self-esteem has to be built among young MSMs growing up in a state of confusion and self-condemnation about their sexual identity. And a cultural space needs to be fostered where men can live with other men, or go through life single without conforming to the societal norm of compulsory marriage and free from any guilt or rejection.

The various MSM support groups are staffed by a combination of Naz personnel and volunteers. Topics of discussion at weekly meetings include: self esteem, feelings of guilt, pressure to marry, gay rights, safer sex practices, and how and where to meet other gay men. While many of these issues are not directly part of Naz's explicit agenda (i.e., to prevent HIV/AIDS), the existence of the support groups is invaluable from an advocacy point of view. Providing a space for these men to meet, talk and feel supported gives Naz greater credibility in the eyes of the MSM community. We believe that a greater degree of rapport with groups such as these makes it easier for us to effectively communicate and carry forward the safe sex message. And we have observed that over the last few years the acceptance of the safe sex message has indeed increased among MSM. And enhancing their ability to access condoms has made a big difference to the community's sense of self-empowerment. The safe spaces afforded to them by the support groups is also giving members of the community the confidence to go in for HIV testing and early self-care.

An offshoot of working with MSM is the Naz-sponsored innovation in condom production and distribution. This again illustrates the principle that advocacy alone unsupported by service provision cannot go very far. When Naz's outreach workers asked MSM if they were using well-lubricated condoms, they were met with derisive laughter. The common reply was, "We would, if we could find them!" The fact – something that we had not realised before – was that well-lubricated condoms suited to MSM sexual activity simply did not exist. Clearly, it did not make sense to advocate a technology that was non-existent. We therefore decided to respond with a service. The result was a series of experiments with different brands of condoms available in the market. When none of these proved satisfactory, Naz decided to bring to the market its own brand of condoms, produced by a private supplier and available at very nominal price (we found that providing them free resulted in the men not taking the idea seriously). Naz continues to monitor the quality and effectiveness of the product through its outreach work.

Early in our work with MSM, a major concern was how to reach HIV-related information to the women married to men who were having sex with other men. On the basis of our interactions, we discerned that the ease with which several women used MSM terminology for sexual acts suggested that women might actually be familiar with MSM activity; this did not rule out the possibility that they may be aware of this activity even on the part of their husbands. The question, however, was how to get across to them, particularly with knowledge of the risks of HIV transmission. We explored two sets of options. We approached women's groups themselves and NGOs providing services to women, with a view to persuading them to include MSM issues in their outreach work. However, this initiative did not go far. This was still in the early 1990s, when the issue of sexuality itself did not figure prominently in the work of women's groups. The other and more productive route that we followed was to conduct sexuality education in schools and colleges wherever our initiative was welcomed, or where we were able to break down barriers of resistance. Here, the challenge was how to include the complex issue of sexual identity and related issues of personal choice, societal norms, Indian values, etc.

By 1996, both the Ford Foundation and the MacArthur Foundation were ready to support work on women's sexuality and on HIV, including MSM. For Naz, which had hitherto been ploughing its own lonely furrow, this provided the opportunity to experiment with cutting-edge work with MSM. One of our first moves was to set up an HIV/AIDS clinic with additional service provisions for MSM, offering pre- and post-test counselling, testing and treatment and, where possible, referrals. Another initiative was the preparation of MSM-specific material with accurate and useful information pertaining to HIV/AIDS and sexually transmitted infections (STIs), including information about transmission modes and their associated risk factors, non-transmission, risk reduction measures, particularly use of condoms and lubricants, and how to get access to treatment. Collaboration with other NGOs from India, Bangladesh and Sri Lanka led to the development of a training manual for promoting MSM sexual health. This manual was meant to sensitise NGOs and community-based organisations to MSM-related issues, as well as to provide a framework for developing services and programmes for the benefit of MSM. Without advocating either the curtailment of genuine sexual desire or conformity to mainstream values, the manual conveyed the need for responsible sexual behaviour and the means through which this might be possible.

The effort at creating and animating the MSM support groups (referred to earlier) was stepped up. The aim of this effort was to create an environment for resolving issues related to MSM sexual identities and behaviour, so that these men could be at ease with themselves, and alert to their own sexual health. The groups certainly served to provide a sense of community. By the late 1990s, the Naz office had become a hub for MSM groups in Delhi, and a role model for similar groups elsewhere in the country. It also served as a drop-in centre for accurate information on issues concerning sexuality, particularly for this marginalised group, virtually the only one of its kind in the city of Delhi. These developments even inspired the emergence of a lesbian group – Sangini – of middle class English-speaking women. After a few years of shelter under the Naz umbrella, Sangini has now registered itself as an independent body. The men's support groups, however, are presently still hesitant to move out of the Naz fold. But where earlier they had been relatively segregated groups – Hindi-speaking, English-speaking, married men, *kothis* – they have now begun to network with each other and look for common spaces across the class and linguistic divide.

Despite Naz's work, progress has been slow particularly when seen in terms of stemming the tide of HIV infection in the community. This raises the question about the efficacy of Naz's methods of working with this marginalised group, i.e., through building self-help and support groups. One of the lessons seems to be that building self-esteem and peer pressure, and their translation into self and mutual protection, is a long, arduous and slow process. It is often in the intimate environment of the family that MSM experience their earliest forms of abuse and rejection of their sexual identity. This is compounded by stigmatisation by the wider society. All this makes the task of sustaining secondary reference-cum-support groups even more necessary and challenging.

Policy advocacy

A recent initiative by Naz is a national level advocacy campaign for legal reform relating to its core constituency of MSM.

MSM groups have called upon Naz from time to time to provide active guidance and support when they face major civil rights abuses, whether in Delhi or in other parts of the country. The traditional criminalisation of MSM has meant power in the hands of the police to 'punish' homosexuals for their 'unnatural' ways, while subjecting them to extortion and/or sexual assault while in police custody. Paradoxically, the 'targeting' of 'high risk' groups by government in the context of HIV/AIDS has heightened MSM visibility (in a way similar to sex workers) and, therefore, stepped up their victimisation by law and order agencies, often on the excuse that they were found in possession of condoms or of sexuality-related printed materials, materials that MSM support groups need to use as part of their HIV/AIDS prevention work. Naz is being called upon more and more for the support that it can extend these groups and, in turn, Naz staff and volunteers have grown in the skills required to handle such situations.

The notion that homosexuality is 'unnatural' continues to be deeply embedded in the law, and law enforcing agencies are quick to resort to Section 377 of the Indian Penal Code (IPC), and treat MSM as criminals. This makes national level advocacy for the human rights of MSM a priority with Naz. As long as such laws are in place, progress in the matter of MSM sexual health, particularly in the context of HIV, is bound to be slow and sporadic. Highlighting the outmoded and dubious nature of Section 377 of the IPC and demanding its removal is to assert the principle of equity and respect for diversity, including diversity in sexual choices and identities.

Towards this end, Naz recently initiated a public interest litigation challenging Section 377 of the IPC that criminalises sex between same sex adults. Arguing that in a democratic state, it does not behove the state to interfere in consensual adult sexual activity, the petition filed in the Delhi High Court sought the removal of adult, private, consensual homosexual sex from the ambit of Section 377. The government, however, opposed the plea on the grounds that the public opinion (couched in terms of the "Indian tradition") did not favour a change in the law. The State's argument is that Section 377 needs to be retained in order to be able to prosecute child abusers, the implication here being that all paedophiles are homosexuals. Naz is now in the process of mobilising representatives of gay rights, women's groups, child rights, health and human rights organisations, to work towards a change in the sodomy law, which is a 19th century colonial vestige, long ago abolished in the country of its origin. The coalition – called "Voices Against Section 377" – is also calling for a new law to deal specifically with child sexual abuse. It argues that criminalising homosexual sex has nothing to do with protecting children from sexual abuse, and identifies the State's position on homosexuality as a case of double standards, since the rape of women or of girl children by men has not led the state to question the legality of heterosexuality.

Treatment and care of HIV positive patients

The move by Naz to set up a regular clinic for HIV testing, counselling and treatment was primarily in response to the felt needs of HIV/AIDS patients in general and MSM patients in particular, who face discrimination – fear, stigma, rejection – at the hands of regular service providers. In an ideal world, the Naz clinic would not need to exist. If there were a sufficient number of general practitioners and medical institutions sensitive to and well informed about both HIV and sexuality related issues, there would be no necessity for Naz – a non-medical NGO – to run a medical clinic. Naz hopes that this service provision on its part will double up as an advocacy tool, that it will demonstrate the art of the possible in relation to the care of HIV/AIDS patients, and lead to open sharing, discussion and strategising within the medical community of how the ongoing needs of HIV/AIDS patients might be met, eventually resulting in many more clinics like the one at Naz.

That eventuality, however, is still a long way away. At the present juncture, Naz finds itself pushed along a path of expansion, with little end in sight. The efforts at advocacy and outreach by Naz have kept up a steadily growing demand for the clinic's outpatient services of testing, counselling of the patient and family, advice on nutrition care of the patient, treatment for opportunistic infections, and anti-retroviral therapy (ART) where advisable. True to its mission, Naz provides these services to anyone who asks for it, MSM and non-MSM. Several patients come from distant regions of the country in a state of acute sickness, and even many of the local patients go through periods of serious sickness when they are unable to take care of themselves. The clinic, therefore, soon expanded into a care home with 20 beds, with additional accommodation for carers to stay until the patients are better, and the carers have learnt how to look after them once they are back home.

As AIDS deaths increase in number, the survivors – almost always widowed, abandoned or destitute women and orphaned children – often find that they are HIV positive themselves. Most lack economic support and are often without shelter, having been thrown out of their homes once the male 'breadwinner' is no more. Under these circumstances, the Naz care home becomes their home. Here, homeless survivors, positive patients and the staff of the care home – some of the latter HIV positive themselves – live together. Naz supports the education of the orphaned children – nearly 20 of them at this point in time – in private schools in the vicinity of the care home. There is complete confidentiality about their HIV status. In the convivial atmosphere of the care home, complete with pets and extra curricular activities like karate and art lessons for the children and family-like picnics, all residents have assured access to nutritious food, regular monitoring of their health status, and ART when necessary. Deaths occur here, too, and are mourned within the family-like atmosphere of the care home.

Making a major impact on attitudes within the medical community continues to elude Naz, despite its many efforts. Besides the hospital-based training workshops mentioned earlier,

Naz also solicits the involvement of medical interns in its clinic and care home. The aim is to initiate these young members of the medical community into HIV/AIDS care and, hopefully, over time, build a cadre of doctors specialising in HIV/AIDS treatment. However, medical colleges in the city of Delhi have shown reluctance to send their interns to the Naz clinic. And HIV is still not an area of choice for young urban medical students. There is still a considerable fear about handling HIV/AIDS patients. Sensitisation to HIV/AIDS issues in medical training does not include any education about sexuality. And, the notion that homosexuality is 'unnatural' continues to govern medical practice, leading practitioners to either contemptuously reject MSM patients who approach them, or treat them with electric shocks in order to 'cure' them of their 'unnatural' tendencies.

But idealistic doctors do respond to Naz's advertisements. And Naz helps in their capacity development through a variety of modes. It sponsors them for specialised training at reputed HIV/AIDS medical centres in the NGO sector, such as YRG CARE (Chennai) and Christian Medical Centre (Vellore). It also has an e-mail tie-up with an infectious diseases specialist in the U.S. who updates the interns on anti-retroviral therapy (ART), engages them in continuous learning, and helps monitor the therapies at the Naz clinic and care home. Naz also enjoys goodwill among a number of specialists in mainstream hospitals in the city of Delhi who offer free services in their private clinics to patients referred by Naz, and who make visits to the care home in times of emergency.

Based on its finding that it is almost always men who access its clinic services, Naz has been advocating actively with prevention-of-mother-to-child-transmission (PMTCT) centres to send their positive women to the Naz clinic for timely treatment, counselling and follow up. The ratio of men to women outpatients at the Naz clinic is now slowly changing as a result of these efforts.

To further ensure that more women come forward for testing and treatment, Naz began a home-based programme two years ago. This intervention has several objectives. It was initially begun as an outreach programme to follow-up clinic attendees. Through a team of outreach workers consisting of a counsellor and a nurse, the programme seeks to create a day-to-day support base for patients at the level of the household. In view of the stigma attached to HIV, this outreach team is camouflaged as a TB team. TB is a common disease in poor urban settlements in the country, that does not attract undue curiosity also due to the already ongoing TB Control (DOTS) Programme. This intervention by Naz is also an attempt to advocate the need for early testing and treatment, and self care; it has been Naz's consistent observation that patients – due to a combination of fear and ignorance – come to the clinic only when they are already very sick. A third important objective is to get across the idea that women ought to come forward for testing and treatment.

Women suffer from several disadvantages. They are overworked, health care for them is a low priority within the household budget, and they can lay claim to little emotional support when going through a course of treatment, particularly if it calls for rest and good nutrition. Naz encourages sick women patients to come and stay at the care home for up to a month if necessary, to facilitate their healing. This enables close supervision of their treatment, and their access to nutritious food. It is also Naz's way of demonstrating their value as individuals. Naz's observation has been that patients in general – and women in particular – get better care within their households after they return from a stint at the care home. The reasons are more than one. Patients and carers get a hands-on experience of what constitutes good quality care within a home environment. Also, the absence of segregation in the care home between positive and uninfected persons has a demonstration effect on such patients and their relatives, which diminishes prejudice. HIV positive women who have received treatment at the Naz care home also become advocates, visiting the homes of other patients in their communities currently receiving treatment, and sharing their experiences with them. This creates confidence among the patients, their families and in the neighbourhood at large. This recent intervention is enabling Naz to expand its work into the communities in which its patients are resident. It also strengthens HIV positive people's capacity to negotiate acceptance for themselves within their homes and in the world outside.

The way forward

Today Naz finds itself in an ever-expanding circle of concerns, of which the growing demand for humane and quality care is rapidly becoming the most paramount. This implies greater effort at resource mobilisation, a daunting task given that at present it is a daily struggle to simply break even. The testing, treatment, care and rehabilitation components, particularly, call for large resources. Most donors, however, prefer to support advocacy and prevention efforts rather than treatment and care. Naz's position is that prevention and care cannot be separated from each other, and that advocacy and prevention must be accompanied by service provision, particularly when there is a growing pool of HIV positive persons who are becoming sicker, and the number of persons dying of AIDS is on the increase. In the early phases of Naz's work, there was significant donor agency support; but as we moved towards care and treatment, this support has diminished considerably. Our principal costs are rent (for the care home), food for its inmates, and costs of running the clinic, which include testing and administering ART and other drugs. The revenues that we are able to generate through our training programmes have been an abiding source of support that has given us some measure of both independence and flexibility. As another strategy for achieving relative sustainability, we have invested two large donations in the purchase of land in the heart of Delhi city and construction of a care home with a 20-bed ward, which will also house the outpatients' clinic, office and periodic training programmes. We are also in the process of widening our donor base to include not only the private Foundations and other institutional charities but also individuals, through the 'Friends of Naz', a scheme under which individuals in their personal capacity donate Rs. 1,000 per year and pledge a long-term commitment to continue this support, knowing that it would go into meeting the costs of medicines and nutrition for positive patients.

It is crucial for Naz to become financially sustainable, given its larger mission of protecting people from and bringing care to those affected by this stigmatising and alienating disease, and enabling them to live normal and dignified lives within their families and communities. Its mission is to demonstrate to larger mainstream funding and implementing agencies that this is an achievable and affordable goal. Towards this end, Naz continues to work to change attitudes within the medical community, raise the level of commitment among medical professionals to provide quality treatment for positive patients, and support NGOs to take up HIV/AIDS work.

Persons and groups affected by HIV are rapidly becoming among the most disenfranchised in the country. Naz sees itself, above all, as an organisation committed to the struggle for social justice for them. Among Naz's priorities is the commitment to working with other groups for legal reform so that marginalised groups – such as MSM – hitherto outside the pale of mainstream society, are not discriminated against by law enforcing agencies and at service centres. With few NGOs willing to come forward to work with MSM despite the growing availability of international funds for HIV work, Naz's identification with this marginalised group also remains among its long-term commitments.

Building empowerment, self-esteem, self-protection and rights is a long and slow journey, and one that presupposes several enabling conditions. The leitmotif of Naz is to actively work to unleash those processes that can result in the creation of those enabling conditions.

SECTION SIX

Legal Approaches to HIV/AIDS

An Overview

The significance of legal approaches is that they are importantly and closely linked to the notion of citizens' rights or entitlements that is fundamental to a democracy. Rights become realities only when individuals and groups claim them, and the legal recognition of a right allows this process to take place. Over and above the application of existing laws and, as in India, the Fundamental Rights guaranteed to all citizens under the Constitution, new social issues may throw up challenges which need to be addressed, either through new interpretations of existing laws, or through the formulation of new laws. HIV/AIDS is one such social issue.

When health is described in terms of 'rights' rather than simply needs, it does two things: it upholds the democratic principles of social justice, equity and non-discrimination in the protection of health; and, it holds governments accountable for making health provisions and services available to citizens, without excuses of financial constraints or discriminatory priorities.

A 'human rights' approach to health broadens health issues beyond the domain of clinical medicine and puts the individual at the centre. It treats the rights of the individual as sacrosanct, but also balances this in relation to the public good. In the actual steering of this balancing process, the human rights approach provides for open and public debate, and the participation of affected groups. Thus, 'human rights' refers essentially to *processes*, which, through their universal application, strive to achieve the greatest public good.

Today, several international instruments to which India is a signatory, lay down universally-recognised human rights standards. These standards may be all-too-easily dismissed as so much rhetoric, but they are the result and expression of the aspirations of continuously-unfolding movements for social change and social justice by a wide spectrum of variously disenfranchised groups and the NGOs who work on their behalf. While the Constitutions and legal systems of individual countries enshrine rights to which the governments of those countries are accountable, human rights instruments offer frameworks for extending such accountability to private corporations and international agencies, as well, both within and across countries. Among the greatest contributions of the human rights approach is that it empowers groups to advocate for legal reforms, i.e., the formulation of humane laws applicable across all groups in society.

Nowhere has the notion of 'rights' as 'human rights' become more poignant than in its application to HIV/AIDS-related health policies and interventions, legal and otherwise. The reason is that in the case of no other disease before it – other than leprosy – have stigma and discrimination deprived so many people of their rights to dignity, health care, employment and security of life as in the case of HIV/AIDS. Ignorance and fear about causes and routes of HIV transmission, and irrational discrimination against 'immoral' or 'illicit' sexual behaviour, sexual orientation and HIV status, may spawn demands for laws to legitimise such discrimination. And widespread societal discrimination – to which judges, too, may be victim – may influence the nature of judgements. In order that nothing impinges on a person's equality in the eyes of the law – not his/her sexual behaviour or orientation, or his/her HIV status whether as litigant or witness – it is important that judges and lawyers learn enough about HIV/AIDS so that they can respond with sensitive application of statute law and general legal principles. A society in which cases of discrimination are effectively challenged in court and lead to progressive judgements, fosters an environment for the advance of both the law and the quality of life of its citizens.

It is part of the same argument that calls for the removal of HIV/AIDS from criminal sanctions. HIV/AIDS is not curable and nor is there any vaccine for protection against it. Prevention through modifications in sexual behaviour is the only means of coping with the spread of the epidemic. Rather than criminal sanctions which use threat and punishment, it is education, compassion, and empowerment that can, over time, bring about enduring behaviour change. Two of the groups that are most vulnerable to HIV are sex workers and people of alternative sexual orientation, notably men who have sex with men. Both these groups are currently governed by criminal laws that are in complete violation of their human and fundamental rights. The laws enable the police and law enforcement authorities to harass them and marginalise them even further with no impact whatsoever on the larger social problem of trafficking, for instance. Such harassment has become more acute since the advent of HIV/AIDS. The result is the even further marginalisation of these groups and their greater isolation from any societal structures that offer education or health care. HIV/AIDS has spurred a movement by these groups and their allies for the repeal of the laws that criminalise them and for equal citizenship rights with the rest of society. As one of the most eloquent advocates for the legal rights of positive people, Justice Michael Kirby of South Africa puts it, the "paradox of HIV/AIDS" is that it is the rights of minorities, i.e., affected populations and those most at risk, that must be protected in order to prevent the spread of the epidemic. The rights of those in society at large can be safeguarded only when the rights of those at risk of HIV are protected. It is by integrating vulnerable minorities and HIV infected persons into mainstream society that the HIV epidemic can be contained. For all of the above, legal approaches have to go hand in hand with advocacy – among lawyers and judges, among health care workers, among the police and law enforcement agencies –, so that these groups become more aware of the nature of HIV and are thus less influenced by irrational responses coming from the rest of society.

In the last several years since the onset of the epidemic in India, legal approaches to the violation of positive people's rights have involved the interpretation of the principles contained in common law and application of the Articles enshrined in the Constitution of the country. The freedoms contained in the Constitution cover a very wide variety of rights. The three most important and interrelated areas of rights in the context of the HIV/AIDS epidemic are: discrimination, consent and confidentiality, and all come under the broad umbrella of Article 21 or the right to life and liberty.

Under the Constitution all citizens of the country are entitled to non-discriminatory treatment. However, this right tends to be violated on grounds of a person's perceived or real HIV status in relation to employment, health care, education and other services that the person may access. Arbitrary testing of employees to confirm HIV status, or mandatory testing of all job applicants that bears no relation at all to the person's fitness to carry out the functions relating to the particular job and resulting in dismissal, non-refusal of a job or marginalisation of the employee within the organisation, are all instances of discrimination. Denial of school admission to children – either themselves HIV positive or born to positive parents – who are otherwise fit, or their removal from school when they pose no threat of transmission to others is, again, tantamount to discrimination and denial of life opportunities to the children concerned. Denial of treatment to positive patients, whether in the private or public sector, amounts to the most direct threat to their right to life.

A basic right of all persons in the context of HIV is the right to informed consent and voluntary testing of their HIV status. This is accompanied by the right to pre-test and post-test counselling. This arises out of HIV's identity as an infection with far-reaching personal and social implications. The HIV test, therefore, unlike any other diagnostic procedure, must be strictly in consonance with the principle of individual autonomy which is enshrined in the fundamental right to life and personal liberty under Article 21 of the Constitution.

Allied to this right is the right of the person to protection from disclosure of his/her HIV status, i.e., confidentiality. Although initially, the 'isolationist' approach was resorted to, i.e., public disclosure of a person's HIV status and his/her isolation in the name of protecting the rest of the population, the terrible stigma, discrimination and often brutal violence against positive persons arising out of such a policy (often driving the victims to suicide) and the public health effect of driving the infection underground, have led to the right to confidentiality being upheld as one of the most critical rights in the context of HIV. The private good arising out of respecting a person's confidentiality is now seen as equivalent to protecting the public good, namely, preventing the further spread of the infection by driving it underground. While this right to confidentiality can be creatively interpreted to vest in Article 21 and its guarantee of the right to personal liberty and privacy, it requires much clearer articulation within the framework of the law.

Most of the legal and human rights violations suffered by positive persons arise out of lack of knowledge in society at large about the means of transmission and about the disease in general. Within health care settings – which are one of the most crucial services accessed by positive persons – discrimination, stigma and violation of rights to confidentiality and autonomy arise from health workers' fear of possible infection, and this fear in turn arises out of poor infrastructural provisioning and training, particularly in terms of universal precautions. Universal precautions consist of: hand washing before and after patient contact, use of gloves before touching body substances, of waterproof aprons if there is likelihood of coming into contact with body substances and of mask and goggles to prevent the splashing of blood into the eyes, placing used needles in sharps containers rather than recapping them, putting all hospital wastes into plastic bags, and segregating all soiled linen in laundry bags. Although the chances of transmission of the HIV virus in health care settings are extremely low, the observance of these precautions can fully protect health care workers from even accidental contamination due to blood, mucus, pus or other body substances of HIV positive patients. Universal precautions are universally advisable also because they raise the general standards of hygiene and quality of care in hospitals. The recognition of the right of all health care workers to universal precautions, and the allied right to post-exposure prophylaxis (PEP) in the event of any accidental infection, can act to remove some of the discrimination that HIV positive patients encounter in health care settings.

One of the first legal instruments in the country to sanction discrimination on the basis of HIV status was the Goa Public Health (Amendment) Act which legitimised testing for HIV without consent, public disclosure of HIV status, imprisonment and quarantine, and unfair dismissal from employment. The challenging of this act by human rights lawyers marks a watershed in the long and ongoing struggle to uphold the legal rights of those affected by HIV/AIDS.

The following chapter gives an account of the efforts of such a group of lawyers – the Lawyers Collective – to deal with the social impact of HIV/AIDS infection. Covering virgin ground and spanning a wide range of interventions that include fighting individual cases, conducting advocacy workshops for judges and lawyers, raising awareness about the disease and HIV positive people's legal rights among the entire spectrum of stakeholders, conducting regular monthly information-sharing meetings for legal, advocacy and medical NGOs and for members of the public and raising issues for national debate through journal articles, the Lawyers Collective remains the country's premier legal NGO in the field of HIV/AIDS. On the basis of its study of HIV/AIDS legislations in other countries and its intense and systematic nation-wide consultations, it has framed a comprehensive draft legislation on HIV/AIDS at the request of the Government of India, that is due to be placed before the Parliament.

Meeting the Unmet Legal Needs of Positive People

The Lawyers Collective HIV/AIDS Unit

ANAND GROVER

The Lawyers Collective was set up in Bombay (now known as Mumbai; the two names are used interchangeably in this chapter) 25 years ago by my colleague, Indira Jaising and I, with the mission of giving legal advice, doing legal aid cases, doing free legal work in run-of-the-mill cases and, most importantly, concentrating on public interest cases involving major legal or constitutional issues or affecting large numbers of persons.

Our decision to follow this career path was influenced by several factors. The New Left in Western Europe and the law centres movement in England had had a marked impact upon us. As opposed to the traditional Left which viewed the law and the legal establishment – courts, judges and lawyers – as oppressive tools of the capitalist State, the New Left believed that there was room even in capitalist societies for using the law as a tool to correct the structural imbalances that work against the poor and the working class. The law centres movement recognised that although courts viewed adversaries as equals, justice was denied to the poor and to marginalised groups because they lacked the resources – the most crucial being the high price of legal services – to take full advantage of the judicial process. The law centres endeavoured to facilitate access to the legal apparatus for the poor and the marginalised sections of the population through provision of legal services to these groups. The Indian situation, with the majority of its population belonging to the ranks of the poor, presented to us a strong rationale for a service along these lines. The national Emergency of 1975-76 had just been lifted and interventions based on law had played a progressive role in keeping open democratic spaces; this to us demonstrated that the law had a critical function in moving social movements in the direction of a more vibrant democracy. Further, the Indian Constitution's provision for Fundamental Rights allowed every person to move the High Courts and Supreme Court and challenge not only any State action that violated any of the Fundamental Rights, but also to strike down any statute on the same grounds, or even any Constitutional amendment for that matter. This vested immense powers in the courts of the country, and we believed that this could potentially be used to benefit the majority of citizens.

Early beginnings

Our first step was to form a loose group called Workers' Law Centre. The industrial city of Bombay – our home base – with its largest concentration of workers in the country seemed to present the perfect opportunity to meet the 'unmet legal needs of the disadvantaged, poor and marginalised'. We were reasonably familiar with the labour movement in Bombay and had good contacts among working class organisations in the city. However, we soon realised that we were making a wrong move. The legal needs of the organised working class and its movement were already being well met all over the country. The trade unions had highly developed litigation skills at their command; in fact, some of the stalwarts practising labour law in Bombay belonged to the trade union movement itself. Besides, contrary to our expectation, the organised trade union movement was not interested in taking up issues for the other poorer sections of the society.

We saw the need to shift our focus from the organised labour class to those who were at a far greater disadvantage in terms of the quality of life, access to public goods and services, disaster management, gender, caste and class. We also decided to formalise our group by registering it under the 'Societies' and the 'Public Trusts' Acts. It was now re-christened as the Lawyers Collective. We were small, had little financial or physical resources and, therefore, consciously kept our initial moves modest. What was encouraging was that our decision to concentrate on public interest litigations proved to be the right one. It was around this time that the Public Interest Litigation (PIL) movement in India was gaining momentum, largely as a result of a series of brilliant judgements delivered on some PIL cases by the then Chief Justice of the Supreme Court of India, Justice P. N. Bhagwati. According to tradition, one could approach a court of law only if one had suffered a legal injury and therefore was an 'interested' party (technically known as 'standing' or *locus standi*). PIL, on the other hand, allowed for others who had "a genuine and sufficient interest" in the issue to move the courts to enforce the Fundamental and statutory rights of others who were unable to access the court of law for reasons of indigence and other disabilities. Justice Bhagwati opined that the adversarial system of justice that was developed in the economically advanced Western countries was inappropriate for Indian conditions as it was based on the assumption of "self-identification of legal injury and the self-selection of remedies". These assumptions did not hold true for the poor in India.

At the Lawyers Collective, we began engaging ourselves in some major public interest cases. They involved diverse and important legal issues relating to housing, livelihood, and environment and the most notable were the Bombay pavement dwellers case, the Bombay hawkers case and the Bhopal gas disaster case. The HIV/AIDS-related cases are the latest in the series. In none of these PILs did we charge fees, but subsidised the work of the Collective from the money that all of us as members of the team earned in our private practice.

The Bombay pavement dwellers case

Housing in Mumbai is in the vice-like grip of the real estate developers' lobby, and land values in the city are among the highest in the world. Added to this are poor urban planning and archaic laws. As a result, over half the city's population lives in slums and slum-like conditions. Among this population are pavement dwellers: whole families who live in shacks made of polythene and hessian sheets, pitched on pavements along the roads, with virtually no access to amenities such as water, toilets and other basic infrastructure. On July 23, 1981 when the monsoon rains were at their height, the then Chief Minister of Maharashtra decided to clear the city of Mumbai of its pavement dwellers, the "eyesore" of the city. Without so much as a notice, the state government authorities with the assistance of the police demolished hutments beginning with those around the city's airport. The dishoused persons and their families were forcibly put into buses and deported far away – presumably in the direction of their "hometowns" – so that they would not be able to return. The People's Union of Civil Liberties – a civil liberties group – filed a writ petition in the Bombay High Court praying that the demolitions be stopped, at least while the monsoons were still in full force. Justice Lentin who heard this petition visited the demolition sites and, moved by the plight of those affected by this action of the State, ordered an immediate stay on the demolition and dislocation drive. This, however, was not with a view to providing any lasting relief for the pavement dwellers; the pavement dwellers were permitted to stay on in their dwellings with the understanding that they would remove themselves from the pavements when the monsoon season ended in the month of October, failing which the same State action – demolition – would be resumed.

The Lawyers Collective used this period of interim relief given to the pavement dwellers to prepare and file a petition before the Supreme Court of India, challenging the demolitions and the requirement of the undertaking to the High Court by the pavement dwellers. The petition was filed under Article 32 of the Constitution of India. The argument that we developed was that it was dire economic necessity that had forced the pavement dwellers to come to Bombay in search of livelihood and, in the absence of alternative housing, make the pavements their abode.

Hence, they could not be evicted in the absence of alternative accommodation. We argued, further, that as long as the State did not provide them with alternatives, they had the right to occupy the pavements. Our intention was not to justify that pavements were appropriate sites for dwellings, or that they be occupied permanently. Rather, it was to force the issue of alternative accommodation for the poorest sections of the population. As a corollary to this we also challenged the constitutional validity of Section 313 of the Bombay Municipal Corporation Act that allowed the structures on the pavements to be demolished.

Legally, the case became a landmark in the annals of Indian law. The petition resulted in the Supreme Court of India's recognition of the 'right to livelihood' as part of the 'right to life' guaranteed under Article 21 of the Constitution of India. This proved to be a significant achievement, as the integration of the concept of 'right to livelihood' with the 'right to life' came to be beneficially used in a number of other cases within India as well as in a few other countries. In terms of the lives of the pavement dwellers themselves, however, I would count the case as a failure. Their lot never improved, and they remain at the mercy of demolition squads even today. The Court held that the right to livelihood could be deprived in accordance with the procedure established by law, which is what the Bombay Municipal Corporation Act was. But here, too, there was a positive fallout, in that the issue of housing rights for the poor came to be debated extensively in the process and has since become a part of the national political agenda. The PIL and its aftermath also spawned much litigation on the rights of pavement and slum dwellers, resulting in the Government of Maharashtra ultimately developing a Scheme under which slum dwellers occupying a structure on or before January 1, 1995 are entitled to alternative accommodation provided by the State.

The Bombay hawkers case

The textile sector – the backbone of Mumbai city's industrial structure – was hit hard in the late 1970s, both due to economic recession and change in the product mix. Several textile mills in Mumbai closed down, and the bulk of factory workers were rendered unemployed. The ranks of informal sector workers swelled. In the absence of other avenues of employment, and given the exorbitant property prices that put investment in setting up regular shops for trading way beyond the reach of these 'displaced' workers, they took to hawking or vending goods on the streets and roads for their own survival, resulting in an estimated hundred thousand hawkers on the streets of Mumbai. The Bombay Municipal Corporation Act provided for only 15,000 licensed hawkers in the city; under this provision others were refused licences even when they applied for them. As unauthorised vendors, therefore, the hawkers were regularly subjected to harassment from officials of the civic body as well as the police; they lived and worked under the constant threat of their tiny stalls being demolished and their goods seized. The Union organising them at that time – the Bombay Hawkers Union – approached us for a solution to their problem. We took up their case and approached the Supreme Court of India, arguing for restraint on demolition and for grant of licences to the hawkers. Our plea was that the right to hawk was a part of the Fundamental Right to carry on a trade, occupation and business under Article 19 (1) (g) of the Indian Constitution, a right that could only be reasonably restricted by the law. Not granting licences at all constituted an infringement of that Fundamental Right.

In a significant judgement, the Supreme Court upheld our plea. It held that hawking was indeed a part of the Fundamental Right to carry on a trade or business granted by the above-mentioned Article of the Constitution, and could only be reasonably restricted by law. Although the civic authority was keen on keeping the hawkers from vending food items, the Court permitted hawkers to sell food as well (cheap food bought from street hawkers is the staple for thousands of the poor and working class in Mumbai). The Supreme Court even suggested that proof of any kind of levy or charge collected by the civic body from the hawkers could be a surrogate for a licence.

The Bhopal gas disaster case

On the early morning of December 3, 1984, deadly fumes and gases containing the poisonous methyl isocyanate (MIC) escaped from the Union Carbide plant in Bhopal in the state of Madhya Pradesh. The gases that spread over the major part of Bhopal city killed over 3,000 persons and injured and maimed in diverse ways another 100,000 to 150,000. The vast majority of persons, injured or dead, were from the poorer sections of the population, and were thus not in a position to litigate and actualise their rights on their own. The matter was further complicated as the culprit was not only the local company – the Union Carbide India Ltd. – but also the parent company the Union Carbide Corporation in the United States. The latter was accountable as it had overlooked the requirements of stringent safety standards by permitting the design of a defective plant. The debate was on the issue of jurisdiction. Bhopal became thick with American lawyers who opined that the issue could be taken up only in the courts in the U.S., and they were accordingly busy collecting powers of attorney from the victims to file suits back home. Many local lawyers, too, were joining them in this effort.

We at the Lawyers Collective believed that this line of argument was inimical to the interests of the victims. For one, there was no guarantee that the U.S. courts would actually take up the issue. More importantly, here was a splendid opportunity to build Indian legal jurisprudence on the issue of accountability of multinational corporations operating in India. We advanced our arguments to substantiate this thesis – that the battle ought to be fought in India – through the medium of our own journal, *The Lawyers*. Under pressure to act, the Government of Madhya Pradesh set up a Commission of Inquiry, and we participated actively in its efforts. However, within six months, the inquiry was aborted on grounds of patent protection. The Government of India now filed a suit in the Bhopal District Court on behalf of the victims. Appeals, counter appeals and review petitions followed on what ought to be the quantum of compensation to the victims, and the case travelled from the District Court to the High Court and finally to the Supreme Court. There, ambiguous outcomes emerged. A Bhopal Act came into being, victims were declared entitled to compensation, and orders were issued for distribution of these compensatory amounts to the victims. However, for twenty years thereafter the compensations remained undistributed, and the victims of the gas leak never received their just dues. The whole experience of the Bhopal Gas Disaster Case was a disillusioning one for the Lawyers Collective. What we did learn, however, was the limitations of PILs and Courts when faced with the united might of the State and a powerful multinational corporation.

The disturbing aspect of public interest litigations (PILs) has been that they have not, to date, been able to provide tangible gains to the disadvantaged groups for whose benefit they are filed. The crux of the matter, it would seem, lies in the inertia of both the Indian State agencies and the marginalised/disadvantaged groups. Tangible benefits from PILs can accrue only when the persons or groups of persons on whose behalf the PILs are filed organise themselves and push the State machinery to implement the orders from the Courts. There is thus a need in this regard for strong peoples' organisations which can take up this task.

Launching *The Lawyers* and initiating work in HIV/AIDS

For the realisation of the full potential of legal remedies for the benefit of poor and marginalised groups there is need for debate, discussion and advocacy outside the courts as well. We at the Lawyers Collective recognised the need to develop our own ideas and understanding of legal issues and practices of law that had specific relevance to disadvantaged groups, and to put these ideas and concerns across to a larger audience for feedback and support. To this end, in 1986 we launched a monthly journal – *The Lawyers* – which has maintained an unbroken publishing record to date. Bringing out the journal meant learning-by-doing on several fronts such as printing, publishing, marketing and, above all, maintaining a steady flow of contributions to the journal. To some extent, the past issues of the journal serve as markers for the emergence of major legal issues concerning the poor and other disadvantaged groups in India.

It was around this time (1986) that the first case of HIV/AIDS was detected in the southern Indian state of Tamil Nadu. By 1988, the demand for justice for those discriminated against on account of the disease was knocking on our doors here in western India. Brushing aside the scare and the stigma that still continues to deter many health professionals from responding to the needs of positive patients, Ishwar Gilada, a medical practitioner in Mumbai, made HIV/AIDS his own cause. Setting up an organisation – the Indian Health Organisation – for the purpose, he launched a vigorous advocacy campaign to educate people about the disease and prevent unsuspecting persons from falling victim to it. Some time in 1988 he came to me to ask if I would argue on behalf of a person with HIV/AIDS – Dominic D'Souza – who had approached the Goa Bench of the Mumbai High Court for grant of relief. What began for me as a reluctant nod has today become a major area of involvement both for me individually and for the Lawyers Collective as a group.

The Goa Legislature had amended the Goa Public Health Act and introduced, by an Amendment Act, provisions relating to HIV/AIDS. Under the Goa Public Health (Amendment) Act, if the authorities suspected that any person was HIV positive he/she could be mandatorily tested without his/her consent. If found positive, he/she could be quarantined in an institution. From this followed, naturally, breach of confidentiality – his/her name could be compulsorily revealed – and discrimination. This was the first case of a deliberate choice by the State – the Government of Goa in this case – of an isolationist strategy as against an integrationist one. Basically, the response to HIV/AIDS infection all over the world has varied, both within legal and non-legal spheres, between the isolationist and integrationist strategies. These are polar opposites on the issues of testing, confidentiality and discrimination. In the isolationist strategy a person may be tested on suspicion without his/her consent and, on a positive report, his/her confidentiality may be breached and discrimination naturally allowed to follow, resulting in isolation of the person. By contrast, in the integrationist strategy, a person is tested on a voluntary basis after obtaining his/her informed consent. In this instance, his/her confidentiality remains intact and, instead of discrimination and isolation, the person remains integrated within the family, community and society.

On the basis of the Goa Pubic Health (Amendment) Act, the Government of Goa had tested, without his knowledge, the blood of a young and talented person – Dominic D'Souza – when he had donated blood at a blood donation drive. On examination, his blood sample was found to be HIV positive. Without assigning any reasons or informing him about his HIV positive status, the authorities had quarantined him in a disused tuberculosis sanitorium, where he was not allowed to meet or communicate with anyone. Food was thrown at him, as the attendants at the institution seemed terrified of any close physical contact. Dominic had no idea why he was being humiliated in this fashion. His mother filed a *habeas corpus* petition in the Goa Bench of the Bombay High Court for his immediate release. The Government of Goa had relied on the Goa Public Health (Amendment) Act to sustain their action of quarantining Dominic.

Dr. Gilada wanted me to appear before the court on behalf of Dominic. He believed that since I had graduated in biochemistry I would be able to understand and explain to the court the true nature and characteristics of HIV infection. Given my background as a human rights activist, he believed that he might be able to persuade me to take up the case. Initially, I was hesitant to meet this request. Like many others in India, I too believed that HIV/AIDS was a 'Western' problem, whose presence in India was being overblown by 'Western agencies'. I casually asked him about the biochemistry of HIV, and he handed me a great deal of scientific literature. As I read through the material in the course of the night, I found myself being drawn in. Suitably prepared, I went to Goa to argue the case before the Goa Bench of the Bombay High Court.

We amended the original petition and challenged the constitutional validity of the Goa Public Health (Amendment) Act. We argued that the isolationist strategy contained in the Goa Amendment Act did not have a rational basis nor a rational relationship to the objective of the legislation, and we mustered extensive scientific literature to demonstrate the validity of our arguments. We further argued that under the Act there was no opportunity for the person who had tested HIV positive to challenge what had been found against him/her. In the course of the hearings, all aspects of HIV were examined, not least sex and its different practices. The arguments lasted two whole days; however, our efforts did not seem sufficient. Concluding the hearings, Justice Mohta who headed the bench jocularly remarked that not only had he learnt a lot about the law and HIV but also about sex. But the Court rejected our argument against the isolationist aspect of the law, on the basis of a single World Health Organisation (WHO) document that stated that isolation of an HIV positive person may be resorted to in certain circumstances. The Court held that in view of that, the legislature had not acted totally irrationally and that, in any event, it was not for the Court to sit in appeal over the legislature. However, on the issue of the opportunity to the person to challenge his/her ostensible HIV status, the Court held that principles of natural justice have to be read into the statute and that the person has to be given the opportunity to rebut any finding declaring him/her HIV positive.

Following the judgement in the *Lucy D'Souza* case, there was a possibility that the Central Government too might introduce a Bill on the lines of the Goa law. Fortunately, by that time, strong objections were voiced by various civil society groups against the draconian nature of the law as represented by the Goa Amendment Act. International opinion and advice from U.N. agencies, too, were against such laws. Eventually, no such law was introduced by the Union Government of India, and even the Goa Act has not been enforced at all. It does, however, continue to remain on the statute book of that state.

Stepping up HIV/AIDS-related legal work

Dominic was a talented theatre artist and very popular in Goa. On knowing that he was HIV positive, he diverted his talent and energies to fight against discrimination and became particularly active in the international HIV/AIDS arena. Indeed, he was the first Indian HIV positive activist. Inexorably, the infection took its toll, and soon Dominic was reduced to skin and bones. Unexpectedly, one day I was told that he had arrived in Mumbai and was in hospital, and had expressed a wish to see me. I was leaving for Delhi and stopped by to meet him on my way to the airport. He seemed to know that his time was up, but I was yet to realise this. This was my first encounter with a full-fledged AIDS death. Brushing aside my inquiries about his health and welfare, Dominic asked searching questions about the Lawyers Collective and its work. He then asked me if I would promise to continue to work against the discrimination of HIV positive people and fight legal battles on their behalf. This was a totally unexpected question. More as a response to the moment, I said yes, with little thought of what this might mean for me. It was a commitment that was to haunt me for the next four years until the successful conclusion of the Lawyers Collective's first employment discrimination case, *MX v ZY*.

But from then on, on behalf of the Lawyers Collective, I began taking up HIV cases more proactively. The cases, however, were still few and far between, perhaps three or four in a year.

This time around, individual HIV cases were taken with a purpose. On the one hand, there were hardly any precedents to go by, but on the other, there was a great deal of stigma against HIV, and more than reason it was stigma that determined the fate of HIV cases. If we had to do HIV cases, it would need to be with a view to affecting the course of the legal stream. In the uncharted waters of HIV in India in those early days, individual cases had to become signposts and milestones for the journey ahead. This strategy was to pay dividends later when we were asked by the government to draft a law on HIV. In a small way, I also began doing HIV advocacy work. Indeed, the first national level workshop on HIV and legal and ethical issues that was organised by the Lawyers Collective was held in Dominic's home state of Goa in the year 1994. The setting up of the HIV/AIDS Unit at the Lawyers Collective in 1998 was the culmination of that fateful promise to Dominic.

The *MX* case

In 1995, a person working as a casual loader in a public sector corporation approached us for legal aid. He had been working for some time and was short-listed for absorption in a permanent capacity. He was found fit on all counts, including lung function and eyes. However, he was found to be HIV positive. For this reason, the corporation decided against his absorption into its workforce. The corporation sought to sustain its action on a rule which made it mandatory for all recruits to be tested for HIV, and if anyone were found to be HIV positive he/she would not be recruited. We challenged both his non-absorption and the rule on the grounds that they were discriminatory (Articles 14 and 16) and infringed his right to livelihood (Article 21) under the Constitution of India. We also applied to the court to have the name and identity of the worker suppressed from public disclosure. The court allowed the application and the case was then heard as *MX v ZY*.

The court passed a judgment of seminal importance in the HIV/AIDS arena. The opening sentence reads as follows: "Is it permissible for the State, under our Constitution, to condemn a person infected with HIV to virtual economic death before he must eventually meet his death due to the ailment, is the question before us? The question is of great contemporary significance and importance." The Court held that the State could not refuse employment to an HIV positive person if he/she was functionally fit to do the job, he/she did not pose any significant risk to others in employment and customers of his/her employer, and if he/she was qualified to do the job. As *MX* satisfied all the three criteria, the corporation was directed to give him back his job, and the rule in this behalf was struck down as being unconstitutional.

The day the *MX* judgment was delivered was perhaps one of the happiest days in my professional life. Not only had we succeeded in the case, I had also kept my promise to Dominic. As if on a pilgrimage, I went to Dominic's house in Goa. As I wandered through the house, I could feel Dominic's spirit all around me. When I came out I found myself weeping uncontrollably. In a manner of speaking, the ghost of Dominic was now exorcised.

The *MX* judgement set a precedent internationally, and the criteria in *MX* are now universally accepted. In India, however, *MX* applied only to State sector employment, there being no anti-discrimination law applicable in the private sector. The principles, however, were capable of being applied in cases of termination of employment in the private sector.

Setting up the Lawyers Collective HIV/AIDS Unit

The successful conclusion of the Dominic and MX cases, the polemical journal articles in *The Lawyers*, the seminars and workshops that we organised and participated in as part of our HIV/AIDS advocacy work all drew the attention of international donor agencies towards us. Offers of support followed for capacity-building at the Lawyers Collective, and for sustained work relating to the human rights of people living with HIV/AIDS (PLWHAs). Most notable among the donors were the United Nations Development Programme (UNDP), the European Commission, the Swedish International Development Agency (SIDA) and the Ford Foundation.

Within our group we discussed the pros and cons of such funding, assessed our own potential for further work in this direction, and came to the conclusion that we were ready to commit ourselves to expanding our involvement in this sphere of human rights. In essence, this would mean professionalising our services but with the commitment associated with NGOs. By now we were also convinced of the importance of advocacy in the success of public interest issues. Steady funding would provide us with an opportunity both to maintain a link with what was going on internationally and to expand our work in India beyond Maharashtra and Goa. We would now be able to freely participate in seminars, conferences and workshops, conduct training programmes of our own and intensify the advocacy and legal aid activities of the Lawyers Collective. It would also give us an opportunity to plan our work in a systematic manner. The donors required us to submit proposals, giving the justification, scope and work plan.

The HIV/AIDS Unit formally came into existence in 1998, started with a grant from the European Commission. Under the terms of the grant, our key constituency would be HIV positive persons, or Persons Living with HIV/AIDS (PLWHAs), and our focus would be the advancement and protection of their rights. The HIV/AIDS Unit would only take up legal cases if the persons who approached us were positive, i.e., if there was a direct HIV issue involved (this did not preclude us from responding to requests for legal advice or services as long as we did not fund these services from the European Commission grant). What this essentially meant was that we would now have to make a conscious effort to render services to PLWHAs. Fortunately for us, there was already an ongoing effort on the part of a national PLWHA group – the Indian Network of Positive Persons (INP+) – to form state level groups. We resolved to remain a professional service organisation that would render services to PLWHAs and their groups as a priority.

We were aware that the HIV epidemic had already entered the general public from the vulnerable groups, and this had important consequences for our legal strategy. Hitherto, HIV had affected only persons who were most vulnerable, chief among whom were sex workers, their clients, injecting drug users (IDUs) and men having sex with men (MSM). As already highly stigmatised groups in our society, they were not likely to approach the courts on grounds of discrimination due to their HIV status. However, with the epidemic creeping into the mainstream society, non-stigmatised persons were likely to need and access legal services. The two most significant groups from this point of view were workers who were likely to be thrown out of their jobs because of HIV and women who would be increasingly disproportionately affected by HIV. Our analysis was to prove correct. The vast majority of the cases handled by the Unit are of workers discriminated against at the workplace and women who are denied their rights within the marital home or even in their husbands' place of employment.

Advocacy was another activity that we intensified. Persons and groups most vulnerable to contracting the virus – sex workers, women, men who have sex with men (MSM), and injecting drug users (IDUs) – required information and knowledge about their legal rights. The other key group whom we wanted to target for advocacy were health care workers, the first port of call for any positive person accessing a health service. Stigma and discrimination in the health services sector was high, and changing the mindsets of health care workers the need of the hour. People living with HIV/AIDS (PLWHAs) were another obvious candidate for our advocacy services.

We therefore consciously started a process of networking with a wide range of groups with whom and through whom we intended to reach the people that we were going to serve. To begin with we attended meetings of NGOs and PLWHA groups, to let them know that we were available and, importantly, to 'sink roots in the NGO community', so to say. In these gatherings, our legal officers were able to meet potential clients in their own environments and thereby could fully comprehend the myriad problems faced by them and their families. For some groups from amongst us – particularly service providers – these meetings provided a forum for building genuine and mutually beneficial relationships. When a group needed legal work to be done they would call upon us to render the services. If an HIV positive person of our acquaintance was in need of special nutrition or medicine or some other special service, we knew which groups could render those services or could put us in touch with others in a position to help. As a result, an NGO network has developed, whose constituents assist each other in providing services to clients. For us, the meetings also served as advocacy sessions on the issue of rights in the HIV context.

Soon we were conducting regular advocacy workshops with all the stakeholders: health care workers, PLWHA groups, NGOs providing help and care to positive people, community volunteers, lawyers, judges and administrators. In these workshops we emphasised the rights-based approach to HIV/AIDS and discussed issues of consent to testing, confidentiality, discrimination and access to treatment.

The workshops that we organised for the judiciary are worthy of special mention. We had realised early on that there was need to sensitise legal professionals and judges to HIV/AIDS if we had to advance related rights issues through the courts. We were fortunate to get international support in this endeavour. Justice Kirby, senior-most judge of the highest court in Australia, the High Court, and Justice Cameron of the South African Court of Appeal – himself HIV positive – offered to come to India and conduct judicial sensitisation sessions. With their help we conducted judicial workshops in Mumbai, Ahmedabad, Delhi, Kochi, Bangalore and Kolkata. These workshops were attended by High Court judges, the subordinate judiciary and members of the Bar Associations.

Among our other activities was publishing small leaflets for different stakeholders explaining HIV/AIDS-related rights issues in simple and direct ways, and bringing out periodical posters on important aspects. We also started the practice of holding open meetings on the first Thursday of every month. These meetings have been ongoing in the cities of Delhi and Mumbai and have been very successful in bringing the HIV/AIDS community together in these two cities to discuss common issues.

As a result of our varied efforts NGOs, PLWHA groups and even several government bodies have become reasonably well versed in rights-based information on legal and ethical issues, and act as disseminators for the same through their own networks. This has been one of the successes of our Unit. Besides building capacity in others, we have been beneficiaries ourselves; we have been enriched by our vibrant links with the HIV community as a whole, and have grown in our understanding, abilities and energies.

Our aim was to set up offices in Mumbai, Delhi, Bangalore, and Kolkata or Imphal within the five-year tenure of the European Commission grant. This ambition has been realised only partially. Initially, we concentrated on Mumbai. We have been fortunate to have obtained and retained good staff for legal work. This is not a common experience; most good lawyers do not wish to work full-time with NGOs, both because that leaves them with no time for more lucrative private practice and because it is not considered a wise step for career advancement. In Mumbai, in fact, it was a problem to identify and attract the right people for advocacy work. Attrition was high, and it took all of the five years to stabilise this aspect of the work. In Delhi, on the other hand, where we set up an office in the year 2000, it worked the other way round. It has been easy to set up a stable team of advocacy officers, but finding a stable set of legal officers has been a problem. One important reason was the apparent paucity of HIV positive people in Delhi and the lack of HIV positive people's networks, due to which legal work relating to HIV/AIDS was slow to take off. Another reason was the absence of an organised working class movement in the city. If HIV positive persons from among the poor are engaged in informal sector occupations where they are not organised into trade unions, they tend to lack in legal and rights literacy. Hence, very few clients were from a working class background.

People from the armed forces have dominated the client profile in Delhi, making the constituency of clients there very different from the one in Mumbai. There are other differences as well between the two cities, for which I can only hazard explanations. Mumbai's long history of organised working class activism has meant pride among legal professionals in committing themselves to fighting for the rights of the disadvantaged. In Delhi, on the other hand, where political and social issues are to the fore, relatively more people flock to and stay with advocacy-related roles rather than hard core legal ones.

The Bangalore office of the Unit has been set up only as recently as late 2004. As the prevalence of HIV/AIDS is higher in the outlying districts of Karnataka than in the city of Bangalore, our work will focus more on these districts. Moving rights issues beyond the cities into small towns and rural areas – in keeping with the spread of the virus itself – has been a new challenge for us. We have already made a beginning in this direction in Maharashtra, our familiar terrain. Although Mumbai has the highest demand for legal and advocacy services, the districts in the hinterland are now showing an increasing seroprevalence. In conjunction with the Network of Positive Persons in Maharashtra (NMP+), we have begun legal aid and advocacy work in the districts of Pune, Aurangabad, Beed, Parbani, Satara and Sangli, with a legal officer from the Unit visiting every month for advice and legal aid. We are also tying up with local lawyers in these districts to do legal aid work, and building their capacity on HIV/AIDS issues is on our agenda. In Karnataka, we expect that advocacy rather than litigation work would be of greater relevance; we have established links with a number of NGOs who have actually developed alternative dispute resolution mechanisms at the grassroots, and who prefer to use a legal course of action only as the last resort. This has led us to strengthen the advocacy component in our Bangalore office. Our participation in the Affordable Medicines and Treatment Campaign (AMTC) has been the first in this series.

Through our legal work we have been able to establish the applicability of principles laid down in the *MX* case to those cases involving termination of employment within the private sector as well. A notable case was that of *RM* who was terminated from his service in the private sector on account of being HIV positive. He was qualified to do the job, was functionally fit, and did not pose any significant risk to his co-workers. We filed a complaint on his behalf in the Industrial Court in Mumbai under Item 9 of Schedule IV of the Maharashtra Recognition of Trade Unions and Prevention of Unfair Labour Practices Act (MRTU and PULP) Act. Item 9 of Schedule IV of the MRTU and PULP Act provided that "non-implementation of an award, settlement or an agreement" is an unfair labour practice that is actionable. The expression "award, settlement or agreement" has been held by the Supreme Court in the *SG Chemicals* case as being very wide in its connotations, including statutory conditions of service. We also applied for the suppression of identity of the complainant. The Industrial Court granted the order of suppression of identity and finally held in our favour, setting aside the termination and reinstating the workman and, further, granting wages that were lost in the interim period on account of the termination. However, although we were able to win the order in favour of our client, it took a long while to implement it in all respects. We were able to get him reinstated fairly quickly, but getting him his wages retrospectively took an enormous amount of time. That is the problem with litigation, and I believe that it should, therefore, be undertaken only as a last resort. If one can achieve a substantive amount through negotiations, it is a preferable option to litigation. Not only does one persuade employers through a dialogue, one also avoids problems in implementation.

Right to marry suspended and restored

As our advocacy work expanded, we were increasingly called upon to address meetings of different stakeholders. At one of these gatherings I met a young doctor, who told me his heart-rending story and whose case we subsequently took up. He – *Mr. X* as he came to be referred to later in court records – had been employed in the medical services of a north-eastern state of the country. In the course of his service, he was asked to escort the relative of a minister in the state government to a government hospital in one of the southern states where the said relative was to undergo an operation. At some stage during the patient's hospital stay, *Mr. X* was asked if he would be willing to donate blood for the patient to which he readily agreed. Apparently, he tested HIV positive, but was not informed and nor was the finding confirmed. Rather, the hospital did not lose time in disclosing this information to others, and the news quickly reached his colleagues, friends, family and relatives. The operation concluded, the party returned home to the north-east. It was there that *Mr. X* learnt what had happened. He found himself shunned by his colleagues, friends and society at large to the extent that he gave up his secure job and migrated to another state in the country. He had earlier been engaged to be married, but called it off in the light of his HIV status. He now told me that he wished to bring the hospital to book for breaching his confidentiality and disclosing his HIV status to others without even confirming it or first informing him.

On our advice, he filed a consumer complaint in the National Consumer Redressal Forum in Delhi. The Forum passed an order that the matter was not amenable to the jurisdiction of the Consumer Court but it could be appropriately taken up by a civil court. In our opinion the Forum was wrong in passing such an order and we advised him that an appeal by Special Leave Petition ought to be filed in the Supreme Court challenging the Consumer Forum's order declining to exercise the jurisdiction vested in it. To our utter disbelief one morning we saw a report carried by a national daily newspaper that the Supreme Court had suspended the right of an HIV positive person to marry. It was the case relating to *Mr. X*. The Supreme Court had not only given such an order and judgement, it had even allowed the name of the person to be published. The first thing we had to do was to get the name suppressed; it took us nearly a month to get that order. The next thing was to attend tc what the Supreme Court had done. We had approached the Supreme Court on the matter of breach of confidentiality. Since *Mr. X* had himself called off his engagement immediately upon knowing his HIV status, the Supreme Court had overstepped its bounds by making a pronouncement on the matter of his marriage. The only legal route that we now saw for *Mr. X* was to file a review petition in the Supreme Court which would go before the same judges. But he was not interested; he had already suffered great damage, and was completely distraught.

In the meanwhile, taking a cue from the Supreme Court judgment, some persons had started advocating a policy for restricting the right of HIV positive persons to marry. In response, we at the Lawyers Collective HIV/AIDS Unit, in collaboration with several other NGOs, launched a nation-wide Right to Marry Campaign. We organised meetings across the country and emphasised to civil society communities represented by NGOs, positive people's groups and community-based organisations (CBOs) that the restriction on the right of an HIV positive person to marry would only drive the disease underground and would be catastrophic for HIV prevention efforts. Similarly, we were able to persuade some NGOs that the right to marry judgement of the Supreme Court was not only wrong but also unwarranted, and that it needed to be corrected through a legal process. The Right to Marry Campaign became a tool for us to pedagogically educate these wide-ranging groups about the legal process – its positive features as well as some pitfalls – and assure them that it was important not to lose hope in the face of setbacks such as this. The matter was eventually heard by another set of judges who held that in the circumstances of the case there was no warrant for the earlier bench to have suspended the right to marry. However, it took nearly three years to rectify the blunder that had occurred.

· Expanding the scope of the HIV/AIDS Unit

In 2003 when the European Commission grant to the Lawyers Collective came to an end we had no problem in finding new sources of support. The Swedish International Development Agency (SIDA) became our funder. With this shift we also made a significant change to our programme. Whereas earlier we had been obliged to restrict ourselves to legal cases where the persons concerned were HIV positive, we now expanded our portfolio to include people from marginalised communities – sex workers, intravenous drug users (IDUs), men who have sex with men (MSM) – who were not actually HIV positive, but extremely vulnerable to the infection. We are currently in the process of formalising this expanded programme – called the Civil Rights Initiative – first in Mumbai and then in our Delhi and Bangalore offices. We foresee that this will pose new challenges in terms of work culture and tactics.

The rights of sex workers

As part of this enlarged focus, we took a case of sex workers in the city of Surat in Gujarat who had been driven out of their homes. Almost five centuries ago during the period of Moghul rule this colony of sex workers had taken up residence here, in the days when this area was outside Surat city limits. With the growth of the city down the centuries, this colony had become part of the city. It was now prime property and middle class residents wanted the sex workers out while real estate developers were keen on acquiring the land. Backed by both these groups and politicians the police attempted through daily harassment to evict the sex workers from their dwellings and prevent them from re-entering. The sex workers came out to protest, organising rallies, pickets (*dharnas*) and fasts. When none of this worked they came to us. We approached the Gujarat High Court, praying that they be allowed to re-enter their homes. The State argued that the sex workers used their homes as brothels which, as per the law, was a criminal activity. Hence, they could not be allowed to re-enter. We pointed out that denying them entry into their own homes was a violation of their rights under Article 21 of the Constitution. If their homes were indeed brothels, the State would need to follow the procedure specified under the Immoral Traffic (Prevention) Act, and not resort to indirect methods not contemplated in the law. The judges continued to hold that the dwellings in question were brothels not homes and our petition was dismissed; but the judges advised the State to look into the problem and come up with some solution. The sex workers did not lose heart and persisted with their demands through their collective organisation on the grounds that their staying together was imperative to facilitate HIV-related services for their own well-being. We have recently learnt that their persistence has paid off and that the government has offered them alternative accommodation within the city itself.

The rights of men who have sex with men (MSM)

We have learnt that it is not the success or failure of legal remedies alone that is critical. Collective organisation and self-generated advocacy around legal issues can become powerful sources of sustenance for vulnerable groups. In a similar case to the one above, the Naz Foundation India – an NGO working with men who have sex with men (MSM), among other vulnerable groups – approached us as they wished to challenge the anti-sodomy law, Section 377 of the Indian Penal Code (IPC). Naz was finding it difficult to provide HIV-related services to MSM communities due to constant harassment of these communities by the police. They rightly deduced that Section 377 IPC was the underlying cause of the harassment and impediments to their ongoing work. According to the settled position in law, Naz had sufficient interest in the issue and bona fide reason to challenge the constitutional validity of the provision. We drafted a petition and filed it in the Delhi High Court. Most of the judges it came up before were of the opinion that the matter required detailed consideration. They accordingly issued Rule – a step that courts take when they consider the matter serious enough to be decided on a full hearing – and also issued notice to the Attorney General of India (since the constitutional validity of a law was being challenged). However, when the matter came up before the Division bench headed by the then Chief Justice, the petition was dismissed on the ground that, as Naz was not personally aggrieved – there being no case under Section 377 IPC filed against them – the petition was not maintainable. This went against the whole development of the public interest litigation (PIL) law in India. A review petition against that order was also dismissed.

Legally, Naz now had two options before it: to file a review, or to file an appeal in the Supreme Court. When we had originally filed the petition, we had done so like traditional lawyers, i.e., through negotiation between us and our client Naz. However, now we were unable to arrive at a consensus on what the next step ought to be. By this time, community participation around the legal proceedings had become intense. Since the outcome of any decision would have affected the community of MSM all over India, there was criticism that we had not consulted the community before filing the petition in the first place. Like traditional lawyers, we had apprehensions about how we would accommodate a wide-scale consultation in drafting and filing the petition. However, we bowed to the better wisdom of the community, and decided to pro-actively involve the community in the decision about the petition. Representatives of interested groups met, and it was their decision that we should file a review petition. As expected – very rarely do judges entertain review petitions – the review petition was dismissed. The question now came up whether we should pursue an appeal on the issue of the maintainability of the petition in the Delhi High Court or, alternatively, file a petition in the High Court of another state in the country. There were different opinions within the community on this. The real worry was that the Supreme Court might, as in the Right to Marry case, simply take up the issue on its merits and decide the case, against which there would then be no appeal. We again had a major and effective consultation with the representatives of the community. It is always difficult even in the best of circumstances to get groups to come together, and my colleague Vivek Divan played an invaluable role in this. Despite differences, the community was able to take a collective step in an informed and participatory manner and, importantly, the discussions about which road to take were of a high quality. The final decision at the end of the consultation was to file an appeal to the Supreme Court only on the issue of whether the Delhi High Court was correct in finding that Naz Foundation India did not have the standing to file and maintain a PIL, and thereby dismissing the petition. Now the matter is in the Supreme Court of India, which recently issued notice to the government to remand the matter back to the Delhi High Court to decide the matter on merits.

The right to treatment using anti-retroviral (ARV) drugs

Although HIV is still incurable, by the mid-nineties it had become treatable due to the advent of triple combination anti-retroviral therapy (ART). However, the costs of ART were prohibitive until late into the year 2000. It was only when the Indian pharmaceutical company Cipla Ltd. announced the reduced price for ARVs that prices across the world plummeted from over USD 15,000 to just USD 400 per annum, with the downward trend still continuing. The cost of medicines has been critical for HIV positive persons, particularly in poor countries. For instance, in the last three years, nearly 30 of the HIV positive clients with us have died on account of the fact that they were unable to afford HIV anti-retroviral therapy, and were unable to get onto the free government programme that began on April 1, 2004.

Realising that affordability and accessibility to medicines and drugs in general and to ARVs in particular was a major issue, a group of NGOs launched the Affordable Medicines and Treatment Campaign (AMTC) in 2001. We campaigned for the availability of ARVs free of cost to those who needed them and could not afford them. We explained that HIV positive persons have a right to live and ARVs are the only means for them to survive. We explained that ARVs were available not only in developed countries but also in developing countries, such as Brazil, free of charge to those who needed but could not afford them. We also pointed out that it was ironic that Indian pharmaceutical companies were busy exporting ARVs to Latin America and Africa while positive people in India were dying. We argued that it was a great opportunity for Indian firms, with their ability to make available drugs produced at the cheapest rates in the world, to give a better life to the HIV positive population of their own country. Ultimately, we were able to convince the government that there was a real need to initiate the ARV rollout programme. Backed by the WHO's *3 by 5* initiative (three million HIV positive persons on ART by 2005 across the world), the Indian Government announced that free ARVs would be available from April 1, 2004, with the aim of having 100,000 HIV positive people on ARVs by 2005. The combinations of drugs and simplified fixed doses would be the ones recommended by the WHO.

Although the initiative was lauded by all concerned, progress has been woefully inadequate. As of February 1, 2005, only 2,700

HIV positive persons have been put on the government's ART programme. There are a number of shortcomings. To cite just two, the Government of India gives no financial support for the programme; all support comes from international Funds such as the Global Fund to Fight AIDS, Tuberculosis and Malaria. And, the infrastructure for drug delivery is skeletal and faulty, so it is anybody's guess how the government will achieve its target. The challenge for the AMTC is to be able to push the government to first keep to its targets and then go beyond them.

The government, through the President of India, promulgated the Patent Ordinance in December 2004, amending the Patents Act. This was later replaced by the Patent Bill. Both the Ordinance and the Bill introduced by the current government were identical to that issued by the government that was earlier in power. Amending the Patents Act was an obligation under the Trade Related Intellectual Property System (TRIPS), but proposed amendments went beyond TRIPS such as to seriously compromise the accessibility and affordability of medicines in general and ARVs in particular in the country. We in the AMTC intensified our campaign, pointing out the shortcomings in the proposed amendments and particularly lobbying in relation to four areas: patentability criteria, pre-grant opposition, compulsory licensing and export to underdeveloped countries. We were able to get some amendments made particularly on patentability and pre-grant opposition. However, India has not taken full advantage of the flexibility in TRIPS. That battle is still an unfinished one.

Keeping the perspective right

It is a matter of some satisfaction that the HIV/AIDS Unit at the Lawyers Collective has progressed considerably in its aim of putting together a professional legal services group in different parts of the country to work for the rights of those affected by HIV/AIDS. Our advocacy work is streamlined, and our networks are wide and deep. We also remain fierce about retaining our independence and autonomy.

In addition to what we have already set out doing, our main tasks over the next few years will be getting the HIV Bill through Parliament, conducting a successful campaign on the Patents debate, and ensuring that the ARV rollout is working properly. Although most people believe in the rights-based approach, there is a concerted attack on this approach from the medical establishment. This has been reinforced by the routine testing protocols being followed by the WHO in the *3 by 5* initiative for the ART rollout around the world. There is great need not only in India but across the world for persons working in the health field, from a human rights perspective, to gather empirical evidence to substantiate the rights-based approach.

The HIV/AIDS epidemic is now spreading rapidly into other areas in India. The Andhra Pradesh Network of Positive People, for example, has 25,000 HIV positive persons as its members. There is a need for legal services there as well as in Manipur, Nagaland and Tamil Nadu (which together with Maharashtra and Karnataka constitute the six high prevalence states as assessed by NACO). There are several challenges before our Unit. Would we be able to develop our capacity to provide the required legal services all over the country, or at least in the six high prevalence states? If we do expand, would we be able to sustain the compactness of and equal opportunities for growth for all within the group, values that are important to us? Would we be able to sustain the quality of our services that our clients expect of us? So far, we have grown at a pace that we find comfortable, and accelerating it may or may not suit our inherent genius. But can the HIV epidemic wait for the luxury of our pace? Alternatively, how would we go about seeding new groups around the country that could work alongside us? How would NGOs such as ours meet the challenge of recruiting dedicated and talented young lawyers to work in an environment that calls for commitment to egalitarian and non-competitive values and willingness to forego the highly remunerative alternatives within the legal profession and in the burgeoning corporate sector? These are going to be some of the main challenges for us in the future. Time alone will tell whether we are up to overcoming them successfully.

Index